Allergy Primer for Primary Care

Editor

MICHAEL A. MALONE

PRIMARY CARE:
CLINICS IN OFFICE PRACTICE

www.primarycare.theclinics.com

Consulting Editor
JOEL J. HEIDELBAUGH

September 2016 • Volume 43 • Number 3

ELSEVIER

1600 John F. Kennedy Boulevard • Suite 1800 • Philadelphia, Pennsylvania, 19103-2899

http://www.theclinics.com

PRIMARY CARE: CLINICS IN OFFICE PRACTICE Volume 43, Number 3
September 2016 ISSN 0095-4543, ISBN-13: 978-0-323-46264-8

Editor: Jessica McCool
Developmental Editor: Colleen Viola

Primary Care: Clinics in Office Practice (ISSN: 0095–4543) is published quarterly by Elsevier Inc., 360 Park Avenue South, New York, NY 10010-1710. Months of issue are March, June, September, and December. Periodicals postage paid at New York, NY and additional mailing offices. Subscription prices are $225.00 per year (US individuals), $434.00 (US institutions), $100.00 (US students), $275.00 (Canadian individuals), $491.00 (Canadian institutions), $175.00 (Canadian students), $345.00 (international individuals), $491.00 (international institutions), and $175.00 (international students). Foreign air speed delivery is included in all *Clinics* subscription prices. All prices are subject to change without notice. POSTMASTER: Send address changes to *Primary Care: Clinics in Office Practice*, Elsevier Periodicals Customer Service, 11830 Westline Industrial Drive, St. Louis, MO 63146. Customer Service Health Sciences Division, Subscription Customer Service, 3251 Riverport Lane, Maryland Heights, MO 63043. **Customer Service: 1-800-654-2452 (U.S. and Canada); 314-447-8871 (outside U.S. and Canada). Fax: 314-447-8029. E-mail: journalscustomerservice-usa@elsevier.com (for print support); journalsonlinesupport-usa@elsevier.com (for online support).**

Reprints. For copies of 100 or more, of articles in this publication, please contact the Commercial Reprints Department, Elsevier Inc., 360 Park Avenue South, New York, NY 10010-1710. Tel. 212-633-3874; Fax: 212-633-3820; E-mail: reprints@elsevier.com.

Primary Care: Clinics in Office Practice is covered in *MEDLINE/PubMed (Index Medicus)* and *EMBASE/Excerpta Medica, Current Contents/Clinical Medicine, and ISI/BIOMED.*

Contributors

CONSULTING EDITOR

JOEL J. HEIDELBAUGH, MD, FAAFP, FACG
Clinical Associate Professor, Departments of Family Medicine and Urology; Clerkship Director, Department of Family Medicine, University of Michigan Medical School, Ann Arbor, Michigan; Ypsilanti Health Center, Ypsilanti, Michigan

EDITOR

MICHAEL A. MALONE, MD
Department of Family and Community Medicine, Penn State Milton S. Hershey Medical Center, Associate Professor, Penn State College of Medicine, Hershey, Pennsylvania

AUTHORS

AYESHA ABID, MD
Department of Family and Community Medicine, Penn State Milton S. Hershey Medical Center, Hershey, Pennsylvania

HADI BHURGRI, MD
Gastroenterology Fellow, Rutgers University, New Jersey Medical School, Newark, New Jersey

DEEPA BURMAN, MD, FAAFP, FAASM
Faculty; Director of Resident Research and Scholarly Activity; Director of Primary Care Sleep Medicine, University of Pittsburgh Medical Center (UPMC) McKeesport Family Medicine Residency, McKeesport, Pennsylvania

KATHERINE CURCI, PhD, NP
Department of Family and Community Medicine, Penn State Milton S. Hershey Medical Center, Hershey, Pennsylvania

NIDHI DHAWAN, MD
Department of Family & Community Medicine, Penn State Milton S. Hershey, Penn State College of Medicine, Hershey, Pennsylvania

SHEYLA PAMELA ESCOBEDO CALDERON, MD
Peruvian Society of Family and Community Medicine, Federico Villareal National University, Lima, Peru

SAMUEL N. GRIEF, MD, FCFP, FAAFP
Associate Professor, Department of Family Medicine, University of Illinois at Chicago, Chicago, Illinois

KRISTEN GRINE, DO
Assistant Professor, Department of Family and Community Medicine, Penn State University College of Medicine, Penn State Hershey Medical Group, State College, Pennsylvania

SARA HALVERSON, MD
Assistant Professor, Department of Family Medicine, Loma Linda University, Loma Linda, California

AMY HAYS, MD
Assistant Professor, Department of Family and Community Medicine, Penn State Hershey Medical Group, State College, Pennsylvania

LORENZO HERNANDEZ, MD, MS
Resident Physician, Department of Family Medicine, Mayo Clinic, Jacksonville, Florida

SKYE HESTON, MD
Department of Family Medicine, Penn State Milton S. Hershey Medical Center, Hershey, Pennsylvania

TIFFANY HILL, MD
Department of Family & Community Medicine, Penn State Milton S. Hershey Medical Center, Penn State College of Medicine, Hershey, Pennsylvania

ECLER JAQUA, MD
Department of Family Medicine, Loma Linda University, Loma Linda, California

HASAN A. KAKLI, MD
Department of Family & Community Medicine, Penn State Milton S. Hershey Medical Center, Hershey, Pennsylvania

HOBART LEE, MD, FAAFP
Assistant Professor, Department of Family Medicine, Loma Linda University, Loma Linda, California

REGINA MACKEY, MD
Department of Family Medicine, Loma Linda University, Loma Linda, California

MICHAEL A. MALONE, MD
Department of Family and Community Medicine, Penn State Milton S. Hershey Medical Center, Associate Professor, Penn State College of Medicine, Hershey, Pennsylvania

VAN NGUYEN, DO
Assistant Clinical Professor, Department of Family Medicine, Loma Linda University, Loma Linda, California

SARAH PAPALIA, MD
Resident Physician, Department of Family Medicine, Mayo Clinic, Jacksonville, Florida

GEORGE G.A. PUJALTE, MD, FACSM
Assistant Professor, Department of Family Medicine, Mayo Clinic College of Medicine, Mayo Clinic, Jacksonville, Florida

JUAN QIU, MD, PhD
Associate Professor, Department of Family and Community Medicine, Penn State University College of Medicine, Penn State Hershey Medical Group, State College, Pennsylvania

EFREN RAEL, MD, FAAAAI
Clinical Director, Sean N. Parker Center for Allergy and Asthma Research, Stanford University, Stanford, California

TIMOTHY D. RILEY, MD
Department of Family & Community Medicine, Penn State Milton S. Hershey Medical Center, Hershey, Pennsylvania

SAMIULLAH, MD
Assistant Professor of Medicine, Division of Gastroenterology, University of Missouri, Columbia, Missouri

LAUREN SIMON, MD, MPH, FAAFP
Associate Clinical Professor, Department of Family Medicine, Loma Linda University, Loma Linda, California

MADHAVI SINGH, MD
Assistant Professor, Department of Family and Community Medicine, Penn State Hershey Medical Group, State College, Pennsylvania

UMAIR SOHAIL, MD
Gastroenterology Fellow, Division of Gastroenterology-Hepatology, University of Missouri, Columbia, Missouri

KONSTANTINOS TOURLAS, MD
Resident Physician; PGY-3; Chief Resident, University of Pittsburgh Medical Center (UPMC) McKeesport Family Medicine Residency, McKeesport, Pennsylvania

ABDUL WAHEED, MD, FAAFP
Assistant Professor, Department of Family & Community Medicine, Penn State Milton S. Hershey Medical Center, Penn State College of Medicine, Hershey, Pennsylvania

JASON RAYMOND WOLOSKI, MD
Department of Family Medicine, Penn State Milton S. Hershey Medical Center, Hershey, Pennsylvania

Contents

Allergic diseases are common in outpatient primary care. Allergy testing can guide management to determine allergy as a cause of symptoms and target therapeutic interventions. This article provides a review of common methods of allergy testing available so that physicians may counsel and refer patients appropriately. Immediate-type hypersensitivity skin tests can be used for airborne allergens, foods, insect stings, and penicillin. Radioallergosorbent testing can be used to evaluate immediate-type hypersensitivity. Delayed-type hypersensitivity or patch-type skin tests are used in patients with suspected contact dermatitis.

Food allergies are common and seem to be increasing in prevalence. Preventive measures have become far more evident in the public arena (schools, camps, sports venues, and so forth). Evaluation and management of food allergies has evolved such that primary care practitioners may choose to provide initial diagnostic and treatment care or refer to allergists for similar care. Food allergies, once considered incurable, are now being diminished in intensity by new strategies.

An adverse drug reaction relates to an undesired response to administration of a drug. Type A reactions are common and are predictable to administration, dose response, or interaction with other medications. Type B reactions are uncommon with occurrences that are not predictable. Appropriate diagnosis, classification, and entry into the chart are important to avoid future problems. The diagnosis is made with careful history, physical examination, and possibly allergy testing. It is recommended that help from allergy immunology specialists should be sought where necessary and that routine prescription of Epi pen should be given to patients with multiple allergy syndromes.

Allergic asthma refers to a chronic reversible bronchoconstriction influenced by an allergic trigger, leading to symptoms of cough, wheezing, shortness of breath, and chest tightness. Allergic bronchopulmonary aspergillosis is a complex hypersensitivity reaction, often in patients with asthma or cystic fibrosis, occurring when bronchi become colonized by *Aspergillus* species. The clinical picture is dominated by asthma complicated by recurrent episodes of bronchial obstruction, fever, malaise, mucus production, and peripheral blood eosinophilia. Hypersensitivity pneumonitis is a syndrome associated with lung inflammation from the inhalation of airborne antigens, such as molds and dust.

Insect bites and stings are common. Risk factors are mostly associated with environmental exposure. Most insect bites and stings result in mild, local, allergic reactions. Large local reactions and systemic reactions like anaphylaxis are possible. Common insects that bite or sting include mosquitoes, ticks, flies, fleas, biting midges, bees, and wasps. The diagnosis is made clinically. Identification of the insect should occur when possible. Management is usually supportive. For anaphylaxis, patients should be given epinephrine and transported to the emergency department for further evaluation. Venom immunotherapy (VIT) has several different protocols. VIT is highly effective in reducing systemic reactions and anaphylaxis.

The purpose of this article is to review the current available material pertaining to atopic dermatitis, contact dermatitis, urticaria, and angioedema. This article focuses on each disease process's clinical presentation, diagnosis, and management. Although atopic dermatitis and contact dermatitis are similar, their development is different and can affect a patient's quality of life. Urticaria and angioedema are also similar, but the differentiation of the two processes is crucial in that they have significant morbidity and mortality, each with a different prognosis.

In last 30 to 40 years there has been a significant increase in the incidence of allergy. This increase cannot be explained by genetic factors alone. Increasing air pollution and its interaction with biological allergens along with changing lifestyles are contributing factors. Dust mites, molds, and animal allergens contribute to most of the sensitization in the indoor setting. Tree and grass pollens are the leading allergens in the outdoor setting. Worsening air pollution and increasing particulate matter worsen allergy symptoms and associated morbidity. Cross-sensitization of allergens is common. Treatment involves avoidance of allergens, modifying lifestyle, medical treatment, and immunotherapy.

PRIMARY CARE:
CLINICS IN OFFICE PRACTICE

ISSUE OF RELATED INTEREST

Immunology and Allergy Clinics of North America
August 2016 (Vol. 36, Issue 3)
Severe Asthma
Rohit Katial, *Editor*
Available at: http://www.immunology.theclinics.com/

THE CLINICS ARE AVAILABLE ONLINE!
Access your subscription at:
www.theclinics.com

PRIMARY CARE:
CLINICS IN OFFICE PRACTICE

FORTHCOMING ISSUES

December 2016
Hematologic Diseases
Maureen M. Okam and Aric Parnes,
Editors

March 2017
Primary Care of the Medically Underserved
Vincent Morelli, Roger Zoorob, and
Joel J. Heidelbaugh, Editors

June 2017
Integrative Medicine
Deborah S. Clements and Melinda Ring,
Editors

RECENT ISSUES

June 2016
Psychiatric Care in Primary Care Practice
Janet Albers, Editor

March 2016
Obesity Management in Primary Care
Mark B. Stephens, Editor

December 2015
Primary Care Dermatology
George G.A. Pujalte, Editor

ISSUE OF RELATED INTEREST

Immunology and Allergy Clinics of North America
August 2016 (Vol. 36, Issue 3)
Severe Asthma
Rohit Katial, Editor
Available at: http://www.immunology.theclinics.com/

THE CLINICS ARE AVAILABLE ONLINE!
Access your subscription at:
www.theclinics.com

Foreword
"Lifesavers"

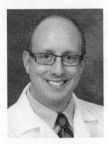

Joel J. Heidelbaugh, MD, FAAFP, FACG
Consulting Editor

I've thought very hard about this, but I don't ever remember any of my classmates in school having life-threatening allergies, much less even a mild food allergy. Maybe that's because I didn't hear or ask about them, but somehow serious allergies were never on my radar. This ignorance later on became extrapolated to my adult life, assuming that the people I'm around everyday didn't have any worrisome allergies, and that these were only rare conditions that you read about or see on test questions.

One typical day several years ago, I was busy in my office, teaching my medical students, behind in my patient schedule, and bearing the average daily amount of work stress. My wife was home with our 5- and 3-year-old daughters, eating lunch and enjoying their day, when I received a series of frantic text messages sequentially over a few seconds. My wife had shared her salad with our oldest daughter, and within a few minutes, my daughter was vomiting, crying uncontrollably, and her lips were turning blue. The last text message read, "going to ER now—meet us there!"

After running out of my clinic and miraculously escaping a speeding ticket, I arrived in the ER of our local hospital and ran directly into our daughter's room—and didn't even recognize her. What I saw was a child with a purple face and eyes swollen shut, an oxygen mask, an IV, and a bunch of wires hooked up to monitors—certainly not my blonde-haired and normally energetic princess. While I was visibly panic stricken, my daughter seemed quite calm and professed, "I'm going to be fine Daddy, they gave me some lifesavers!" Somehow, I couldn't make the connection between the popular candy and the treatment of anaphylactic food allergies. Within only a few short minutes, I saw the amazing effects of epinephrine, methylprednisolone, and diphenhydramine reverse the immunologic effects of the toxic pine nuts from the salad and restore my daughter to her normal state. Then, she devoured a Popsicle in world-record time!

Within a few hours, life was back to our "normal" equilibrium. But the very next evening at dinner, we shared my masterful salmon with teriyaki glaze (read: fish plus sesame seeds). What followed was round two of our family allergy nightmare experience,

Prim Care Clin Office Pract 43 (2016) xiii–xiv
http://dx.doi.org/10.1016/j.pop.2016.06.001
0095-4543/16/$ – see front matter © 2016 Published by Elsevier Inc.

which began with a much less severe reaction in our younger daughter that was luckily rapidly reversed by oral diphenhydramine, but provided a much greater, heightened sense of fear in her parents and older sister. After another trip to the ER, countless consultations with allergists, and a stock pile of EpiPens at home and at school, my family is now experts on how to read labels on food packaging, how to interrogate restaurant servers and chefs about potential cross-contamination of food, and how to avoid any of their (known) allergens. And, my daughters still want to know exactly what xanthan gum is....

My wife, a pharmacist of almost 20 years, remains my greatest source of knowledge for all things related to medications and their adverse effects. Much of her job involves the often arduously dreaded "medication reconciliation" for primary care and specialty practices. This leads to many dinner conversations about patients who take more than a dozen drugs and supplements, how they interact, how patients develop allergies versus intolerances to medications, and how to sort all of this out in my daily practice.

This issue of the *Primary Care: Clinics in Office Practice* explores the pathophysiology and immunology behind common environmental and pharmacologic allergies. The first article embraces the challenging task of allergy testing and deftly guides readers through common testing modalities and their limitations. Subtopics within allergy common to our practices are then presented, including insect, environmental, and pharmacologic allergies. An article on allergy immunotherapy helps to distill the finer points of this science to simplify this concept for primary care providers. Systemic conditions affecting pulmonary, gastrointestinal, dermatologic, and otolaryngologic conditions outline the profound multisystem effects of various allergens. Finally, complementary and alternative therapeutic options for treating allergies are explored.

I genuinely thank Dr Michael Malone and his authors for their dedication and impressive efforts in compiling this compendium of articles on the topic of allergy. Creating a volume of high-quality articles on the topic of allergy is no small feat, and this issue will clearly be an invaluable reference for all health care practitioners as the prevalence of allergies increases, and as we become more aware of their potentially life-altering and horrific consequences. Prior to our family's experiences with our children, I didn't understand much about serious allergies, or their potential impact on quality of life. After my own medical education, my knowledge of allergies grew, but this issue has helped to significantly advance my training and to become far more surveillant of potential allergens that we all may encounter.

Joel J. Heidelbaugh, MD, FAAFP, FACG
Departments of Family Medicine and Urology
University of Michigan Medical School
Ann Arbor, MI 48109, USA

Ypsilanti Health Center
200 Arnet Suite 200
Ypsilanti, MI 48198, USA

E-mail address:
jheidel@umich.edu

Preface

Allergy Primer for Primary Care

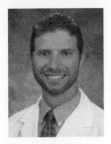

Michael A. Malone, MD
Editor

Primary care physicians are the initial or continuity provider for many patients with allergic conditions. Thus, a quality medical reference for these conditions is necessary. Therefore, I am pleased to present this issue of *Primary Care: Clinics in Office Practice* devoted to allergy-related disorders. The thirteen topics covered in this issue were selected to address conditions that would be of clinical relevance and easily utilized in a busy primary care setting. Each article is set up for quick and practical reference during patient care, including key points and tables that summarize essential information about the allergy topics. Current evident-based guidance on assessment and treatment is included for topics seen in everyday practice, such as food and drug allergies, insect allergies, allergy testing, allergic rhinitis, and allergic dermatoses.

Primary care providers can also improve patient care outcomes for less common conditions encountered in their practice. Therefore, topics such as eosinophilic gastrointestinal disorders have also been in included in this issue for clinical reference. Although each article is set up for quick reference, each topic also provides a thorough overview of clinical presentations, diagnosis, and treatments. I hope you enjoy reading this issue and find it both evidence-based and clinically relevant.

Michael A. Malone, MD
Department of Family and Community Medicine
Penn State College of Medicine
Hershey, PA 17033, USA

2643 Westhampton Terrace
Elizabethtown, PA 17022, USA

E-mail address:
mmalone@hmc.psu.edu

Prim Care Clin Office Pract 43 (2016) xv
http://dx.doi.org/10.1016/j.pop.2016.04.014
0095-4543/16/$ – see front matter © 2016 Published by Elsevier Inc.

primarycare.theclinics.com

Erratum

An error was made in the June 2016 issue of *Primary Care: Clinics in Office Practice* on page 308 in "Eating Disorders in the Primary Care Setting" by Devdutta Sangvai. In the last sentence of the second paragraph, only Table 6 should be cited, instead of Tables 6 and 7.

Prim Care Clin Office Pract 43 (2016) xvii
http://dx.doi.org/10.1016/j.pop.2016.07.013
0095-4543/16

Allergy Testing

Konstantinos Tourlas, MD, Deepa Burman, MD*

KEYWORDS

- Allergy testing • Skin prick testing • Intradermal testing • In vitro allergy testing
- Patch testing • IgE hypersensitivity • Allergen

KEY POINTS

- Allergic diseases are commonly seen in the primary care office setting; indiscriminate battery of allergic testing is not routinely recommended without presence of clinical symptoms.
- Symptomatic patients can undergo allergen specific immunoglobulin E (IgE) testing to help guide allergen avoidance.
- Skin testing can be performed by percutaneous or intradermal route.
- Serum total IgE level measurement is not very helpful, but assays for specific IgE antibodies can be considered in appropriate situations.
- In cases of persistent or chronic allergic rhinitis and allergic asthma, specific allergic testing may be helpful.

INTRODUCTION

Allergic diseases are commonly seen in the primary care setting. More than 50 million Americans suffer from allergic rhinitis. Asthma affects about 20 to 30 million Americans, which in many instances has an allergic component to it.[1] Allergic skin conditions are also prevalent. Primary care physicians need to be comfortable assessing and managing patients with these disorders. Knowledge and appropriate use of allergy testing is an important component of allergic disorder management. Allergy testing can assist in the possible identification of the individual allergen that is involved in the allergic reaction, which in the long run can help to decrease the morbidity and mortality for patients. **Box 1** summarizes the indications of allergy testing. This article focuses on the common tests used in allergy testing.

SKIN PRICK TESTING

The skin prick method is the best initial means for testing individuals who have potential allergies. The procedure involves cleaning the skin with a 70% alcohol solution.

Disclosure Statement: The authors have nothing to disclose.
Department of Family Medicine, University of Pittsburgh Medical Center (UPMC) McKeesport Family Medicine Residency, 2347 Fifth Avenue, McKeesport, PA 15132, USA
* Corresponding author.
E-mail address: burmand@upmc.edu

Prim Care Clin Office Pract 43 (2016) 363–374
http://dx.doi.org/10.1016/j.pop.2016.04.001   **primarycare.theclinics.com**
0095-4543/16/$ – see front matter © 2016 Elsevier Inc. All rights reserved.

> **Box 1**
> **Indications for allergy testing**
>
> - Perennial or seasonal rhinitis
> - Rhinosinusitis
> - Rhinoconjunctivitis
> - Rhinitis with otitis media
> - Suspected food allergy
> - Suspected drug allergy
> - Suspected insect bite or sting
> - Persistent asthma

After that, a concentration of 1 to 10 or 1 to 20 g/L of the allergen is placed on the skin. It is important to ensure that the correct concentration of allergen, as stated in the package insert, is used. It is also important to make sure that each drop has only 1 allergen when attempting to identify an allergy to a specific substance. In certain circumstances, it is acceptable to use multiple allergens (eg, multiple forms of tree pollen).

When performing the test, the drops should be placed at least 2 centimeters apart. Placing the drops closer to each other increases the potential for cross-contamination of the allergens resulting in potential false-positive or false-negative reading of the test. After the drops are placed, a commercial device is used to prick the skin causing the drops of allergen to go underneath the outer layer of the skin. The older method of "scratching" the skin with a needle or other device is rarely used now because it carries a greater risk for systemic reactions, and is more likely to lead to scars or other damage to the skin.[2]

Appropriate controls are important. The test should include both a positive and a negative control to verify that the patient's skin responds appropriately. The positive control is generally a 10 g/L concentration of histamine dichloride. The negative control is generally the identical concentration of glycerinated saline.

A positive test results is a raised wheal on the skin with surrounding erythema. The histamine control normally produces a wheal of at least 3 mm in diameter. If the positive control does not provide a wheal with a 3 mm diameter, it is possible to simply count any wheal 3 mm or greater as a positive.[3] The wheal of a positive test must be of at least the same size or larger than the histamine control.

The measurements for the size occur at 10 minutes for the control, and 15 to 20 minutes for the allergens themselves. A more precise measurement can be done by measuring the fattest and thinnest part of the wheal, and then expressing this as an average.[4] Sometimes, using ink and putting the size of the wheals on a piece of paper is helpful for the purposes of keeping records.

CONTRAINDICATIONS

Overall, allergy skin prick testing is a safe procedure. Rarely, it can cause systemic reactions, such as anaphylaxis. It is important to make sure that individuals are not at a risk for anaphylaxis. Individuals with a high risk for anaphylaxis include those who have uncontrolled asthma and those who have reduced lung function.

Individuals who have experienced anaphylaxis within the previous 30 days are not good candidates for skin prick tests because the tests results may have a false-negative result. Prior anaphylactic shock causes the skin to be unreactive, a condition that lasts approximately 2 to 4 weeks. If the skin test results in a positive test, the results are still accurate and useful for the purposes of diagnosis of an allergy.

If the individual has had anaphylaxis within the past month, it is still possible to perform in vitro testing. This alternative does not have a risk of having false negatives because the free immunoglobulins are generally less affected by recent anaphylaxis.

Individuals with certain skin conditions should not have skin prick tests because these conditions make it more likely to have false positive results. Some of these conditions include dermographism, urticaria (whether acute or chronic), cutaneous mastocytosis, and atopic dermatitis. For individuals who have atopic dermatitis, it is possible to successfully perform the skin test on areas of the skin that are not affected by the condition.

Other reasons not to perform skin tests (relative contraindications) include active angina and cardiac arrhythmias, older adults who are in poor health, and women who are pregnant. These groups are not necessarily at any greater risk for anaphylaxis, but are much more susceptible to the adverse effects of its treatment. Thus, it is not recommended to perform allergy skin tests on those individuals. **Box 2** outlines some contraindications and caution for skin prick testing.

FACTORS THAT AFFECT RESULTS

Beyond the factors that affect whether or not an individual should undergo the allergy testing procedure, there are also a number of factors that affect the actual results of the test. General factors that affect the accuracy of results include the source of the allergen, or the types of skin test devices that the testing individual decides to use.[5–8] For example, contaminants in the allergens may cause false-positive test results. The purity and quality of the sample may not be high enough to cause a positive test result. Thus, these factors need to be considered when analyzing/interpreting test results.

FACTORS THAT AFFECT RESULTS: MEDICATIONS

Individuals undergoing allergy testing should stop taking certain medications. Certain medications are considered perfectly safe and have no effect on allergy testing. The

---

Box 2
Contraindications for skin prick testing

- Individuals at high risk for anaphylaxis
  - History of severe allergic reaction to small amounts of allergen
  - Poorly controlled asthma and reduced lung function
- Anaphylaxis within the last 30 days
- Certain skin condition
  - Dermographism
  - Urticaria
  - Cutaneous mastocytosis
- Relative contraindications
  - Significant cardiovascular disease
  - Frail elderly adults
  - Pregnancy

medications that do not impair skin test results include: leukotriene receptor agonists, many decongestants, beta agonists, inhaled or intranasal glucocorticoids, oral theophylline and cyclosporine.[9–15]

Among the most common medications that people should stop taking before an allergy test include all types of antihistamine medications. This is because antihistamines are designed to help decrease the allergic response and can cause the individual to have a false-negative test. All types of antihistamines should be discontinued including eye drops, nasal sprays, and oral medications. Stopping all antihistamines 1 week or more before administering the skin prick test should be sufficient to prevent any interference.[16–18]

When individuals have certain types of conditions that require the use of glucocorticoids, it is important to make sure that the testing occurs on parts of the skin that has not been treated with those topical agents.[19–21] In addition, certain types of antiimmunoglobulin treatments for asthma, including omalizumab, can decrease skin reactivity for up to 6 months, and it may be better to discontinue the use of these medications for 6 months before performing the skin prick test.[22,23] H_2 receptor blockers are other medications that people should discontinue 48 hours before administering a skin test.[24]

Another class of medications that can have an effect on skin reactivity are tricyclic antidepressants, which may interfere with skin reactivity for up to 2 weeks.[25] Antidepressants may be difficult to discontinue for that period of time, so noting that individuals are on the medications when performing the skin test is important. If the skin test either has a weak result or has a negative result, it may be better to perform an in vitro allergy test versus a skin prick test. Physicians should remember that selective serotonin reuptake inhibitors do not affect skin testing, and using these medications as an alternative may be a reasonable.

The data on topical calcineurin inhibitors show mixed results, but a lot of studies suggest that discontinuing the use of these medications 1 week before performing the skin prick test should be fine. In general, whenever there are medications that may interfere with the results of a skin prick test (**Box 3**), it is possible to perform in vitro testing.

Box 3
Medications affecting skin prick testing results

- H1a antihistamines – stop 1 week before testing
- Antihistamine nasal sprays – stop 3 days before testing
- Antihistamine eye drops – stop 3 days before testing
- Antihistamines used for nonallergic states (ie, promethazine, prochlorperazine) – stop 2 weeks before testing
- Medications used for vertigo/motion sickness or insomnia (ie, meclizine, doxylamine) – stop 2 weeks before testing
- H_2 receptor blockers – stop at least 48 hours before testing
- Topical corticosteroids – testing should be performed on skin that has not been treated
- Tricyclic antidepressants – may need to stop 2 weeks before testing
- Calcineurin inhibitors – stop at least 1 week before testing
- Omalizumab – may need to 6 months before testing

RISKS

For the most part, skin prick testing results in a localized reaction and is a safe procedure that has little to no risk of complications. However, some individuals may have systemic reactions, such as breathing issues. For this reason, the recommendation is to have emergency equipment available, including epinephrine, to handle these possible systemic reactions.

Certain food allergens or latex may present a much higher risk of having systemic reactions as compared with other allergens. Intradermal testing (rather than skin prick testing) is more likely to result in systemic reactions; however, the risk remains low. Thus, skin prick testing is a much better alternative to intradermal testing. It is advisable to test with skin prick testing before testing with intradermal testing to minimize the chance of anaphylaxis or undesirable outcomes.

A prospective study by Bagg and colleagues[26] involving about 1500 participants reported the overall rate of systemic reactions secondary to skin tests to be 3.6%, none of which were severe. Aeroallergens were responsible for the greatest number of systemic reactions, mostly from intradermal testing rather than simple skin prick testing. Anaphylaxis was present in a very small percentage of individuals who underwent prick or puncture testing, although all of these individuals had a history of asthma. Other risk factors for severe reactions include children less than 1 year of age and children who have active eczema. Additionally, children who had asthma were more likely to experience anaphylaxis as compared with children who did not have asthma.[27,28]

Anaphylaxis in adults who have asthma is also exceedingly rare. Generally, with proper preparation it is highly unlikely that anaphylaxis will result in death.[29]

SKIN PRICK: INTERPRETATION OF RESULTS

A positive result of a skin prick test only demonstrates that there is an immunoglobulin (Ig)E-specific antibody present, but it does not necessarily mean that the individual will have symptoms when exposed to that particular allergen. It is important to ensure that the clinical history coincides with the result. If an individual has no clinical history and a positive result, then this could be indicative of subclinical sensitization or it could be a false-positive result. Individuals who are sensitized subclinically can develop symptoms at any point in time.

By contrast, a negative result is much more informative. A negative result means that the individual does not have an immunoglobulin for a particular allergen, which effectively means that the individual will not display symptoms when they are exposed to the particular allergen.[30]

Table 1 shows the grading scale from 0 to 4 that can be used for assisting in the interpretation of skin prick test results; however, a higher grade does not always indicate worse clinical symptoms.

INTRADERMAL TEST

Owing to the issues with the accuracy of the skin prick testing, an alternative is to perform an intradermal test. These tests carry a much greater risk of systemic reactions, including anaphylactic shock; however, the risk remains low.[31] Intradermal testing is more sensitive, and detects immune responses to allergens with much greater accuracy. However, false-positive results are also much more common, which means that these tests are much less valuable to individuals who present without any clinical symptoms.

Table 1 Interpretation of skin prick test results	
Grade	Wheal
0	≤ Negative control
1	1 mm > control
2	2–4 mm > control
3	5 mm > control
4	Wheal with pseudopods

Adapted from Bush RK. Diagnostic tests in allergy. In: Slavin RG, Reisman RE, editors. Expert guide to allergy and immunology. Philadelphia: American College of Physicians; 1999. p. 8.

The technique for administering the test is the exact same as a tuberculin skin test. Thus, a needle is used to inject of 0.02 to 0.05 mL of a 1:500 to 1:1000 weight per volume allergen extract into the skin.[32] It is not necessary to have a positive control if the skin prick test has already shown sensitivity to histamine. If this is not present, however, it may be necessary to inject histamine to demonstrate the same response as the positive control.

Intradermal testing is performed generally after a negative skin prick test.[33–35] This minimizes the risk of an individual experiencing any systemic reactions. The only exception to this is allergies related to insect venom. Venom allergies are more likely to cause death so intradermal tests are preferred, because they are more sensitive.[36,37] Further, it is not advisable to use intradermal skin prick tests for food allergens because higher rates of systemic reactions that have been reported.

The high risk of anaphylaxis as well as the sensitivity of the test means that it is possible to use more dilute concentrations when performing this test. A lower concentration not only decreases the likelihood of systemic reactions, it also decreases the likelihood of a false-positive response.[1] A positive response is defined as either a wheal that is at least 5 mm in diameter; however, a survey done in 2008 showed that 85% of American board-certified allergists were defining at positive result as any wheal 3 mm or greater in diameter than the negative control wheal. In addition, the 2008 practice parameter of the American Academy of Allergy, Asthma and Immunology states that "Any reaction larger than the negative control may indicate the presence of specific IgE antibody." **Table 2** shows the grading scale used for interpretation of intradermal test results.[38]

Table 2 Interpretation of intradermal test results		
Grade	Wheal (mm)	Erythema (mm)
0	<5	<5
±	5–10	5–10
1	5–10	11–20
2	5–10	21–30
3	5–10 or with pseudopods	31–40
4	>15 or with many pseudopods	>40

Adapted from Bush RK. Diagnostic tests in allergy. In: Slavin RG, Reisman RE, editors. Expert guide to allergy and immunology. Philadelphia: American College of Physicians; 1999. p. 8.

False-positive results are more common with intradermal testing, especially for inhalant allergens. Intracutaneous bleeding caused by needle trauma during the administration of the test can be interpreted falsely as a positive result.

IN VITRO TESTING

There are several other possible ways of testing for allergies. One of these ways is testing in vitro for specific IgE antibodies in the blood, such as the radioallergosorbent test and the enzyme-linked immunosorbent assay. This is generally an acceptable way of testing for allergies when an individual cannot undergo intradermal testing or skin prick testing, owing to contraindications or not being able to stop medications. The sensitivity (60%–95%) and specificity (30%–95%) for these tests are much broader than the skin prick tests.[38,39]

This test detects the presence of allergen-specific IgE antibodies in the bloodstream. The presence of these antibodies is sufficient to predict that a person will have an allergic reaction when exposed to the allergen. However, even if there is a high level of antibodies in the blood, this does not always correlate with severity of the allergic response, if any.

The results of the in vitro testing are classified into multiple classes (**Table 3**) to help increase the predictive value of the test. The higher the allergen class in **Table 3**, the greater the level of allergen-specific IgE antibody present. These categories are helpful in predicting whether or not an individual will display symptoms. Asymptomatic sensitization can be seen in some individuals having less than class III and levels greater than or equal to class III are more consistently related to symptoms upon exposure.[40–42] Therefore, the clinical history of the individual, the level of positivity in the result, and the allergen in question, influence the clinical relevance of the results.

Highly positive results (class VI result) and a history of typical allergic symptoms indicate an allergic reaction to that particular allergen. When there is a slightly positive result (class I result), and no past history of symptoms, this generally requires additional testing. A negative test in the presence of symptoms does not rule out an allergy, and it may be best to perform a skin prick test. In cases where individuals have experienced some symptoms, and the potential allergy is life threatening, in vitro testing may be helpful to confirm a negative skin test.[37]

PATCH TESTING

Patch testing is a very specific form of testing used to determine if an individual has suspected allergic contact dermatitis. The general theory behind patch testing is that individuals who are sensitized to a particular antigen will be able to produce an allergic reaction even when a low concentration of the antigen is placed on normal

Table 3 Phadia Immunoglobulin E immunoassay classes		
Class (By Phadia)	Concentration (kIU/L)	Interpretation
0	<0.35	Levels less than class III is generally associated with asymptomatic sensitization. Levels ≥ class III are more consistently related to symptoms upon exposure. The clinical history of the individual, the level of positivity in the result, and the allergen in question, influence the clinical relevance of the results.
1	0.35–0.7	
2	0.7–3.5	
3	3.5–17.5	
4	17.5–50	
5	50–100	
6	>100	

skin. Patch testing is useful in individuals who have dermatitis for unknown reasons, individuals who work in a field that have high occurrences of dermatitis, and/or worsening of a previous stable dermatitis.[43]

To perform the patch test, a physician places a test allergen on the upper back for 2 days (48 hours). After patch removal, the skin is analyzed to determine whether or not there has been an allergic reaction. This initial reading occurs 15 to 60 minutes after taking off the patch, so that the transient erythema caused by patch placement can resolve. It is important to perform a second read; read the patch over the course of days, so that one can distinguish between irritant reactions (reactions that fade) versus true allergic reactions (reactions that persist) versus delayed allergic reactions (reactions that do not appear at the time of patch removal; **Table 4**).[42] Certain reactions fade quickly, like those related to fragrances. Allergies to nickel and corticosteroids occur over the course of days, and having an additional reading after 6 to seven days ensures that these allergies are not missed. Performing the readings at the appropriate intervals helps minimize the risk of false negatives. Day 4 readings seem to be associated with a low number of false-negative reactions.[44]

If a patch test is negative, despite suggestive clinical history of acute contact dermatitis, then a repeated open application test or usage test can be performed.[43] The repeated open application test is performed by applying 0.1 mL of the allergen in question to an area of skin twice daily for up to 28 days or until an eczematous skin reaction develops.[43,45,46] The usage test is performed by having the individual use the allergen in question in his or her everyday real-world conditions. This test tries to reproduce all the factors (ie, sweating, friction, etc) associated with the original dermatitis. The 1 drawback of this test is that it may fail to differentiate irritant from allergic dermatitis.[43]

SUMMARY

A number of tests are available to help physicians in the diagnosis of allergic disease. These tests work by detecting specific IgE antibodies. Skin prick testing is rapid, sensitive, and cost effective. Intradermal testing is generally used in individuals who have had a negative skin prick test when clinical history suggests an allergic reaction. It is preferred as first line in insect venom allergies. In vitro testing should be used in individuals who cannot undergo skin prick testing, or if skin prick testing is unavailable. Patch testing is useful in individuals with allergic contact dermatitis. Performing these tests will allow physicians to help identify the specific allergen involved in an individual's allergic disease. From here, the next steps can be taken in helping patients manage their allergic conditions. **Table 5** summarizes commonly used allergy tests.

Table 4 Interpretation of patch test results	
Reaction Severity	**Result Interpretation**
−	No skin changes – negative reaction
? or +/−	Mild erythema – questionable reaction
+	Erythema, slight infiltration – mild reaction
++	Erythema, infiltration and vesicles – strong reaction
+++	Bullous, ulcerative lesions – extreme reaction

Table 5
Summary of commonly used allergy tests

Types of Skin Testing	Indications	Contraindications	Risks	Key Points
Skin prick testing	Perennial or seasonal rhinitis Rhinosinusitis Rhinoconjunctivitis Rhinitis with otitis media Suspected food allergy Suspected drug allergy Suspected insect venom allergy Persistent asthma	Individuals at high risk for anaphylaxis Anaphylaxis within the last 30 d Individuals with dermographism, urticarial or cutaneous mastocytosis	Low risk for systemic reactions	Rapid Sensitive Cost effective
Intradermal testing	Same as skin prick testing; however, should generally only be done after a negative skin prick test	Same as skin prick testing	Higher rates of systemic reactions; however, this is still very low	Preferred as first line for insect venom allergies Generally performed after a negative skin prick test, if suspicion still high More reproducible and more sensitive
In vitro testing	Used in individuals who cannot undergo skin prick or intradermal testing, owing to contraindications or not being able to stop medications	None	No risk of systemic reactions	Not affected by the medications patient is taking Not affected by skin disease or reliant on skin integrity Wide sensitivity (60%–95%) and specificity (30%–95%)
Patch testing	Used to identify specific allergens in allergic contact dermatitis Individuals with eczematous dermatitis or chronic dermatitis	Do not place patch on noncontact skin or skin with a dermatitis	An irritant or allergic skin reaction may occur at the site of patch testing, including a rash and a burnlike reaction Low risk for anaphylaxis	Performing a second read is important, so that one can distinguish between irritant reactions vs true allergic reactions vs delayed allergic reactions If patch testing is negative, however, history is suggestive of allergic contact dermatitis, then the repeated open application test or usage test can be performed

REFERENCES

1. Schidlow DV, Smith DS. A practical guide to pediatric respiratory diseases. Philadelphia: Hanley & Belfus; 1994.
2. Oppenheimer J, Nelson HS. Skin testing: a survey of allergists. Ann Allergy Asthma Immunol 2006;96:19–23.
3. Adinoff AD, Rosloniec DM, McCall LL, et al. Immediate skin test reactivity to Food and Drug Administration-approved standardized extracts. J Allergy Clin Immunol 1990;86:766–74.
4. Ruëff F, Bergmann KC, Brockow K, et al. Skin tests for diagnostics of allergic immediate-type reactions. Guideline of the German Society for Allergology and Clinical Immunology. Pneumologie 2011;65:484–95 [in German].
5. Carr WW, Martin B, Howard RS, et al. Comparison of test devices for skin prick testing. J Allergy Clin Immunol 2005;116:341–6.
6. Nelson HS, Kolehmainen C, Lahr J, et al. A comparison of multiheaded devices for allergy skin testing. J Allergy Clin Immunol 2004;113:1218–9.
7. Nelson HS, Lahr J, Buchmeier A, et al. Evaluation of devices for skin prick testing. J Allergy Clin Immunol 1998;101:153–6.
8. Dykewicz MS, Lemmon JK, Keaney DL. Comparison of the Multi-Test II and Skintestor Omni allergy skin test devices. Ann Allergy Asthma Immunol 2007;98:559–62.
9. Simons FE, Johnston L, Gu X, et al. Suppression of the early and late cutaneous allergic responses using fexofenadine and montelukast. Ann Allergy Asthma Immunol 2001;86:44–50.
10. Hill SL, Krouse JH. The effects of montelukast on intradermal wheal and flare. Otolaryngol Head Neck Surg 2003;129:199–203.
11. Cuhadaroglu C, Erelel M, Kiyan E, et al. Role of Zafirlukast on skin prick test. Allergol Immunopathol (Madr) 2001;29:66–8.
12. Roches Des A, Paradis L, Bougeard YH, et al. Long-term oral corticosteroid therapy does not alter the results of immediate-type allergy skin prick tests. J Allergy Clin Immunol 1996;98:522–7.
13. Olson R, Karpink MH, Shelanski S, et al. Skin reactivity to codeine and histamine during prolonged corticosteroid therapy. J Allergy Clin Immunol 1990;86:153–9.
14. Spector SL. Effect of a selective beta 2 adrenergic agonist and theophylline on skin test reactivity and cardiovascular parameters. J Allergy Clin Immunol 1979;64:23–8.
15. Munro CS, Higgins EM, Marks JM, et al. Cyclosporin A in atopic dermatitis: therapeutic response is dissociated from effects on allergic reactions. Br J Dermatol 1991;124:43–8.
16. dos Santos RV, Magerl M, Mlynek A, et al. Suppression of histamine- and allergen-induced skin reactions: comparison of first- and second-generation antihistamines. Ann Allergy Asthma Immunol 2009;102:495–9.
17. Devillier P, Bousquet J. Inhibition of the histamine-induced weal and flare response: a valid surrogate measure for antihistamine clinical efficacy? Clin Exp Allergy 2007;37:400–14.
18. Dreborg S. The skin prick test in the diagnosis of atopic allergy. J Am Acad Dermatol 1989;21:820–1.
19. Andersson M, Pipkorn U. Inhibition of the dermal immediate allergic reaction through prolonged treatment with topical glucocorticosteroids. J Allergy Clin Immunol 1987;79:345–9.

20. Pipkorn U, Hammarlund A, Enerbäck L. Prolonged treatment with topical glucocorticoids results in an inhibition of the allergen-induced weal-and-flare response and a reduction in skin mast cell numbers and histamine content. Clin Exp Allergy 1989;19:19–25.

21. Gradman J, Wolthers OD. Suppressive effects of topical mometasone furoate and tacrolimus on skin prick testing in children. Pediatr Dermatol 2008;25: 269–70.

22. Noga O, Hanf G, Kunkel G. Immunological and clinical changes in allergic asthmatics following treatment with omalizumab. Int Arch Allergy Immunol 2003;131: 46–52.

23. Corren J, Shapiro G, Reimann J, et al. Allergen skin tests and free IgE levels during reduction and cessation of omalizumab therapy. J Allergy Clin Immunol 2008; 121:506–11.

24. Kupczyk M, Kupryś I, Bocheńska-Marciniak M, et al. Ranitidine (150 mg daily) inhibits wheal, flare, and itching reactions in skin-prick tests. Allergy Asthma Proc 2007;28:711–5.

25. Rao KS, Menon PK, Hilman BC, et al. Duration of the suppressive effect of tricyclic antidepressants on histamine-induced wheal-and-flare reactions in human skin. J Allergy Clin Immunol 1988;82:752–7.

26. Bagg A, Chacko T, Lockey R. Reactions to prick and intradermal skin tests. Ann Allergy Asthma Immunol 2009;102:400–2.

27. Norrman G, Fälth-Magnusson K. Adverse reactions to skin prick testing in children - prevalence and possible risk factors. Pediatr Allergy Immunol 2009;20: 273–8.

28. Pitsios C, Dimitriou A, Stefanaki EC, et al. Anaphylaxis during skin testing with food allergens in children. Eur J Pediatr 2010;169:613–5.

29. Bernstein DI, Wanner M, Borish L, et al. Twelve-year survey of fatal reactions to allergen injections and skin testing: 1990-2001. J Allergy Clin Immunol 2004; 113:1129–36.

30. Sampson HA. Update on food allergy. J Allergy Clin Immunol 2004;113:805–19 [quiz: 820].

31. Lockey RF, Nicoara-Kasti GL, Theodoropoulos DS, et al. Systemic reactions and fatalities associated with allergen immunotherapy. Ann Allergy Asthma Immunol 2001;87:47–55.

32. Dolen WK. Skin testing and immunoassays for allergen-specific IgE. Clin Rev Allergy Immunol 2001;21:229–39.

33. Lieberman P, Anderson JA. Allergic diseases. New York: Humana press; 2007.

34. Franklin Adkinson N, Bochner BS, Burks AW, et al. Middleton's allergy: principles and practice e-dition. Philadelphia: Saunders; 2003.

35. Proceedings of the task force on guidelines for standardizing old and new technologies used for the diagnosis and treatment of allergic diseases. Washington, DC. June 18-19, 1987. J Allergy Clin Immunol 1988;82:487–526.

36. Georgitis JW, Reisman RE. Venom skin tests in insect-allergic and insect-nonallergic populations. J Allergy Clin Immunol 1985;76:803–7.

37. Strohmeier B, Aberer W, Bokanovic D, et al. Simultaneous intradermal testing with hymenoptera venoms is safe and more efficient than sequential testing. Allergy 2013;68:542–4.

38. Bernstein IL, Li JT, Bernstein DI, et al. Allergy diagnostic testing: an updated practice parameter. Ann Allergy Asthma Immunol 2008;100:S1–148.

39. Williams PB, Dolen WK, Koepke JW, et al. Comparison of skin testing and three in vitro assays for specific IgE in the clinical evaluation of immediate hypersensitivity. Ann Allergy 1992;68:35–45.
40. Sampson H, Ho DG. Relationship between food-specific IgE concentrations and the risk of positive food challenges in children and adolescents. J Allergy Clin Immunol 1997;100:444–51.
41. Sampson HA. Utility of food-specific IgE concentrations in predicting symptomatic food allergy. J Allergy Clin Immunol 2001;107:891–6.
42. Uter WJ, Geier J, Schnuch A. Good clinical practice in patch testing: readings beyond day 2 are necessary: a confirmatory analysis. Members of the Information Network of Departments of Dermatology. Am J Contact Dermatitis 1996;7:231–7.
43. Bourke J, Coulson I, English J, et al. Guidelines for the management of contact dermatitis: an update. Br J Dermatol 2009;160:946–54.
44. Todd DJ, Handley J, Metwali M, et al. Day 4 is better than day 3 for a single patch test reading. Contact Derm 1996;34:402–4.
45. Hannuksela M, Salo H. The repeated open application test (ROAT). Contact Derm 1986;14:221–7.
46. Villarama CD, Maibach HI. Correlations of patch test reactivity and the repeated open application test (ROAT)/provocative use test (PUT). Food Chem Toxicol 2004;42:1719–25.

Food Allergies

Samuel N. Grief, MD, FCFP

KEYWORDS

- Food allergies • Anaphylaxis • Desensitization • Oral immunotherapy
- Food challenge • Peanuts • Milk

KEY POINTS

- Food allergies are prevalent, especially among children of all ages, requiring identification and treatment or prevention with medication and education to parents, teachers, and other community leaders.
- Nut and milk allergies are the most common food allergies, thus warranting special attention within the childhood population as well as enhanced safeguards within typical community gathering places (schools, amusement parks, camps, and so forth).
- Food challenge and oral immunotherapy are at the heart of identification and potentially reversing food allergies among affected individuals. Undertaking these therapies requires appropriate preparation and caution.

INTRODUCTION

Food allergies are common. Recent statistics show an increasing prevalence of reported food allergies worldwide.[1–3] Food allergies affect people of all ages, ethnicities and heritage. Varying estimates of prevalence have been reported, however. Food allergies affect approximately 5% of adults and 8% of children.[1,4] Among children ages 0 to 17 years, the prevalence of food allergies increased from 3.4% in 1997 to 1999 to 5.1% in 2009 to 2011.[3]

What Are Food Allergies?

Food allergy "occurs when the body has a specific and reproducible immune response to certain foods."[5] Whether the response is mild, moderate, or severe (anaphylaxis), food allergy is usually an adverse health outcome and should be thoroughly evaluated and addressed by medical professionals.[5] Allergic reactions to foods have become the most common cause of anaphylaxis in community health settings.[6]

Food allergy is often mistaken for food intolerance. When a food product causes irritation or digestive upset anywhere along the gastrointestinal tract, this is labelled an intolerance. Symptoms of food intolerance may include the following:

- Flatulence
- Abdominal cramps

Department of Family Medicine, University of Illinois at Chicago, 1919 West Taylor Street, Suite 143, Chicago, IL 60612, USA
E-mail address: sgrief@uic.edu

Prim Care Clin Office Pract 43 (2016) 375–391
http://dx.doi.org/10.1016/j.pop.2016.04.008
primarycare.theclinics.com
0095-4543/16/$ – see front matter © 2016 Elsevier Inc. All rights reserved.

- Bloating
- Heartburn
- Irritability
- General malaise
- Headaches

Lactose and food additives are the most commonly reported food intolerance.[7]

There are numerous risk factors for food allergies. **Box 1** presents the most common risk factors.

PREVENTION

There is currently no cure for food allergies. Strict avoidance of the food allergen is the only way to prevent a reaction.[15] In 2013, the Centers for Disease Control and Prevention published "Voluntary Guidelines for Managing Food Allergies in Schools and Early Care and Education Programs," which delineates a broad, preventative approach to minimizing allergic reactions among school-aged children.[16] **Fig. 1** outlines a checklist for school officials to use as a template for minimizing food allergy–induced outcomes among children.[16]

The 2008 official statement from the American Academy of Pediatrics regarding allergy prevention states[17]

1. At the present time, there is lack of evidence that maternal dietary restrictions during pregnancy play a significant role in the prevention of atopic disease in infants. Similarly, antigen avoidance during lactation does not prevent atopic disease, with the possible exception of atopic eczema, although more data are needed to substantiate this conclusion.
2. For infants at high risk of developing atopic disease, there is evidence that exclusive breastfeeding for at least 4 months compared with feeding intact cow milk protein formula decreases the cumulative incidence of atopic dermatitis and cow milk allergy (CMA) in the first 2 years of life.

Box 1
Risk factors for food allergies

- Antacid overuse
- Atopy (comorbid atopic dermatitis)
- Dietary fat (reduced consumption of omega-3 polyunsaturated fatty acids)
- Genetics (familial associations, HLA, and specific genes)
- Increased hygiene
- Northern climate
- Obesity (being an inflammatory state)
- Race/ethnicity (increased among Asian and black children compared with white children)
- Reduced consumption of antioxidants
- Season of birth
- Gender (male gender in children)
- Timing and route of exposure to foods (increased risk for delaying allergens with possible environmental sensitization)
- Vitamin D insufficiency[8–14]

Check If You Have Plans or Procedures	Priorities for a Food Allergy Management and Prevention Plan
	1. Does your school or ECE program ensure the daily management of food allergies for individual children by:
☐	Developing and using specific procedures to identify children with food allergies?
☐	Developing a plan for managing and reducing risks of food allergic reactions in individual children through an Emergency Care Plan (Food Allergy Action Plan)?
☐	Helping students manage their own food allergies? (Does not apply to ECE programs.)
	2. Has your school or ECE program prepared for food allergy emergencies by:
☐	Setting up communication systems that are easy to use in emergencies?
☐	Making sure staff can get to epinephrine auto-injectors quickly and easily?
☐	Making sure that epinephrine is used when needed and that someone immediately contacts emergency medical services?
☐	Identifying the role of each staff member in a food allergy emergency?
☐	Preparing for food allergy reactions in children without a prior history of food allergies?
☐	Documenting the response to a food allergy emergency?
	3. Does your school or ECE program train staff how to manage food allergies and respond to allergy reactions by:
☐	Providing general training on food allergies for all staff?
☐	Providing in-depth training for staff who have frequent contact with children with food allergies?
☐	Providing specialized training for staff who are responsible for managing the health of children with food allergies on a daily basis?
	4. Does your school or ECE program educate children and family members about food allergies by:
☐	Teaching all children about food allergies?
☐	Teaching all parents and families about food allergies?
	5. Does your school or ECE program create and maintain a healthy and safe educational environment by:
☐	Creating an environment that is as safe as possible from exposure to food allergens?
☐	Developing food-handling policies and procedures to prevent food allergens from unintentionally contacting another food?
☐	Making outside groups aware of food allergy policies and rules when they use school or ECE program facilities before or after operating hours?
☐	Creating a positive psychosocial climate that reduces bullying and social isolation and promotes acceptance and understanding of children with food allergies?

Fig. 1. Food allergy management and prevention plan checklist. (*From* Centers for Disease Control and Prevention. Voluntary Guidelines for Managing Food Allergies in Schools and Early Care and Education Programs. Washington, DC: US Department of Health and Human Services; 2013.)

3. There is evidence that exclusive breastfeeding for at least 3 months protects against wheezing in early life. In infants at risk of developing atopic disease, however, the current evidence that exclusive breastfeeding protects against allergic asthma occurring beyond 6 years of age is not convincing.

4. In studies of infants at high risk of developing atopic disease who are not breastfed exclusively for 4 to 6 months or are formula fed, there is modest evidence that atopic dermatitis may be delayed or prevented by the use of extensively or partially hydrolyzed formulas, compared with cow milk formula, in early childhood. Comparative studies of the various hydrolyzed formulas have also indicated that not all formulas have the same protective benefit. Extensively hydrolyzed formulas may be more effective than partially hydrolyzed in the prevention of atopic disease. In addition, more research is needed to determine whether these benefits extend into late childhood and adolescence. The higher cost of the hydrolyzed formulas must be considered in any decision-making process for their use. To date, the use of amino acid based formulas for atopy prevention has not been studied.

5. There is no convincing evidence for the use of soy-based infant formula for the purpose of allergy prevention.
6. Although solid foods should not be introduced before 4 to 6 months of age, there is no current convincing evidence that delaying their introduction beyond this period has a significant protective effect on the development of atopic disease regardless of whether infants are fed cow milk protein formula or human milk. This includes delaying the introduction of foods that are considered to be highly allergic, such as fish, eggs, and foods containing peanut protein.
7. For infants after 4 to 6 months of age, there are insufficient data to support a protective effect of any dietary intervention for the development of atopic disease.
8. Additional studies are needed to document the long-term effect of dietary interventions in infancy to prevent atopic disease, especially in children older than 4 years and in adults.

Common Food Allergens

Eight foods or food groups account for 90% of serious allergic reactions in the United States:

- Milk
- Eggs
- Fish (eg, bass, flounder, and cod)
- Crustacean shellfish (eg, crab, lobster, and shrimp)
- Wheat
- Soy
- Peanuts
- Tree nuts (eg, almonds, walnuts, and pecans)[4]

To help Americans avoid the health risks posed by food allergens, Congress passed the Food Allergen Labeling and Consumer Protection Act of 2004 (FALCPA).[16] The law requires that labels must clearly identify the food source names of all ingredients that are—or contain any protein derived from—the 8 most common food allergens, which FALCPA defines as "major food allergens."[18]

Food labels must identify the food source names of all major food allergens used to make the food.[18] This requirement is met if the common or usual name of an ingredient (eg, buttermilk) that is a major food allergen already identifies that allergen's food source name (ie, milk). Otherwise, the allergen's food source name must be declared at least once on the food label in 1 of 2 ways.

The name of the food source of a major food allergen must appear

1. In parentheses after the name of the ingredient.
   Examples: lecithin (soy), flour (wheat), and whey (milk)
   OR
2. Immediately after or next to the list of ingredients in a "contains" statement.
   Example: Contains wheat, milk, and soy.[18]

FOOD ALLERGY SYMPTOMS

A food allergy is typically categorized as mild to moderate or severe based on reaction history (Box 2). Mild-to-moderate symptoms are usually reported as

- Angioedema of the lips, eyes, or face
- Other angioedema
- Coughing

> **Box 2**
> **Allergic symptoms**
>
> *Mild–moderate*
> - Abdominal cramps
> - Coughing
> - Face, tongue, or lip swelling
> - Flushed skin or rash
> - Hives
> - Swelling of the throat and vocal cords
> - Tight, hoarse throat
> - Tingling or itchy sensation in the mouth
> - Trouble swallowing
> - Vomiting and/or diarrhea
>
> *Severe*
> - Difficulty breathing
> - Dizziness and/or lightheadedness
> - Loss of consciousness
> - Weak pulse
> - Wheezing
>
> *Data from* Refs.[5,18,19]

- Other oropharyngeal symptoms
- Eczema
- Flushing
- Hives
- Pruritus
- Vomiting[5]

Severe symptoms mainly include any report of

- Anaphylaxis
- Low blood pressure
- Trouble breathing
- Wheezing

A reaction, including vomiting, angioedema, and coughing, in combination is also categorized as severe.[5]

In general, childhood food allergies to milk, egg, wheat, and soy typically resolve during childhood, whereas allergies to peanut, tree nuts, fish, and shellfish are persistent.[20] There is evidence, however, that resolution rates have slowed for allergies that have been commonly outgrown, such as those to milk, egg, wheat, and soy.[20]

Food allergy severity varies—38.7% of children have a history of severe reactions.[4] Among allergic children, 1 or more food allergies affect a strong minority; 30.4% have multiple food allergies.[4]

Prevalence of food allergies among children is included (**Table 1**).

Table 1
Prevalence of common food allergies according to age group

Age Group	All Allergens (N = 3339)	Peanut (N = 767)	Milk (N = 702)	Shellfish (N = 509)	Tree Nut (N = 430)	Egg (N = 304)	Fin Fish (N = 188)	Strawberry (N = 189)	Wheat (N = 170)	Soy (N = 162)
					Frequency, % (95% CI)					
Prevalence among all children surveyed										
All ages (N = 38,480)	8.0 (7.7–8.3)	2.0 (1.8–2.2)	1.7 (1.5–1.8)	1.4 (1.2–1.5)	1.0 (0.9–1.2)	0.8 (0.7–0.9)	0.5 (0.4–0.6)	0.4 (0.4–0.5)	0.4 (0.3–0.5)	0.4 (0.3–0.4)
0–2 y (n = 5429)	6.3 (5.6–7.0)	1.4 (1.1–1.8)	2.0 (1.6–2.4)	0.5 (0.3–0.8)	0.2 (0.2–0.5)	1.0 (0.7–1.3)	0.3 (0.1–0.4)	0.5 (0.3–0.7)	0.3 (0.1–0.5)	0.3 (0.2–0.4)
3–5 y (n = 5910)	9.2 (8.3–10.1)	2.8 (2.3–3.4)	2.0 (1.7–2.5)	1.2 (0.8–1.6)	1.3 (1.0–1.7)	1.3 (0.9–1.7)	0.5 (0.3–0.8)	0.5 (0.3–0.8)	0.5 (0.3–0.7)	0.5 (0.3–0.7)
6–10 y (n = 9911)	7.6 (7.0–8.2)	1.9 (1.6–2.3)	1.5 (1.2–1.8)	1.3 (1.1–1.6)	1.1 (0.87–1.4)	0.8 (0.6–1.1)	0.5 (0.3–0.7)	0.4 (0.3–0.5)	0.4 (0.3–0.5)	0.3 (0.2–0.5)
11–13 y (n = 6716)	8.2 (7.4–9.0)	2.3 (1.9–2.8)	1.4 (1.1–1.8)	1.7 (1.3–2.1)	1.2 (1.0–1.6)	0.5 (0.4–0.8)	0.6 (0.4–0.8)	0.4 (0.3–0.6)	0.7 (0.5–0.9)	0.6 (0.4–0.8)
≥14 y (n = 10,514)	8.6 (7.9–9.3)	1.7 (1.4–2.1)	1.6 (1.3–1.9)	2.0 (1.7–2.5)	1.2 (0.9–1.5)	0.4 (0.2–0.5)	0.6 (0.4–0.9)	0.4 (0.3–0.6)	0.3 (0.2–0.4)	0.3 (0.2–0.4)
P	.0000	.0001	.0504	.0000	.0000	.0000	.1045	.7700	.0089	.0509

Prevalence among children surveyed with food allergy

All ages (N = 3339)	—	25.2 (23.3–27.1)	21.1 (19.4–22.8)	17.2 (15.6–18.9)	13.1 (11.7–14.6)	9.8 (8.5–11.1)	6.2 (5.2–7.3)	5.3 (4.4–6.3)	5.0 (4.2–6.0)	4.6 (3.8–5.6)
0–2 y (n = 469)	—	22.2 (17.4–27.8)	31.5 (26.6–36.8)	7.5 (4.7–11.9)	5.4 (3.6–8.1)	15.8 (12.0–20.4)	4.0 (2.3–6.9)	7.5 (5.2–8.2)	4.0 (2.2–7.2)	4.2 (2.7–6.5)
3–5 y (n = 539)	—	30.3 (25.8–35.3)	22.1 (18.3–26.5)	12.9 (9.7–16.9)	14.3 (11.1–18.2)	13.7 (10.5–17.6)	5.7 (3.8–8.6)	5.5 (3.6–8.2)	5.0 (3.2–7.7)	5.1 (3.3–7.8)
6–10 y (n = 847)	—	25.5 (22.0–29.5)	19.6 (16.6–23.0)	17.1 (14.0–20.6)	14.3 (11.6–17.5)	11.1 (8.6–14.3)	6.2 (4.5–8.5)	4.8 (3.4–6.9)	5.0 (3.5–7.1)	4.0 (2.6–6.2)
11–13 y (n = 584)	—	28.1 (23.7–32.9)	17.7 (14.2–22.0)	20.4 (16.8–24.7)	15.2 (12.0–19.2)	6.6 (4.4–9.9)	7.0 (4.8–10.1)	4.6 (3.1–6.8)	8.2 (5.9–11.2)	6.9 (4.7–10.0)
≥14 y (n = 900)	—	20.2 (17.0–23.7)	18.4 (15.3–22.1)	23.8 (20.1–27.9)	13.4 (10.7–16.6)	4.1 (2.9–5.9)	7.2 (5.2–9.8)	4.9 (3.3–7.3)	3.3 (2.1–5.0)	0.3 (0.2–0.4)
P	—	.0050	.0001	.0000	.0010	.0000	.4646	.4486	.0174	.1296

Common food allergens are those reported with a frequency of n >150.

From Gupta R, Springston EE, Warrier MR, et al. The prevalence, severity and distribution of childhood food allergy in the United States. Pediatrics 2011;128(1): e13; with permission.

SPECIFIC FOOD ALLERGIES
Nut Allergies

Peanut allergy is the most common cause of food-induced anaphylaxis.[21] Exposure to peanuts can occur in various ways.

Direct contact
- The most common cause of peanut allergy is eating peanuts or peanut-containing foods. Sometimes direct skin contact with peanuts can trigger an allergic reaction. This situation may occur at school, arranged outings, or special occasions or in public.

Cross-contact
- Cross-contact is the unintended introduction of peanuts into a product. It is generally the result of a food being exposed to peanuts during processing or handling. Manufacturers are required by law to label foods that may have been processed in a factory where peanuts have been handled or available.[18]

Inhalation
- An allergic reaction may occur if inhaling dust or aerosols containing peanuts, from a source such as peanut flour or peanut oil cooking spray. It behooves individuals with severe peanut allergies to cleanse and prepare their cooking environment accordingly.[21]

Suffice it to say that eating foods outside a controlled environment for any individual with peanut allergies requires vigilance and education. Many improvements to safeguarding the environment for individuals with severe peanut allergies have been made, especially in restaurants, sports and recreational centers, and camps, among others.[22–24]

Peanut allergy risk factors include the following:

Age
- Food allergies are most common in children, especially toddlers and infants. With age, the digestive system matures, and the body is less likely to react to food that triggers allergies.

Past allergy to peanuts
- Some children with peanut allergy outgrow it. Even if they seem to have outgrown peanut allergy, however, it may recur.

Other allergies
- If already allergic to one food, there may be increased risk of becoming allergic to another. Likewise, having another type of allergy, such as hay fever, increases the risk of having a food allergy.

Family members with allergies
- There is increased risk of peanut allergy if other allergies, especially other types of food allergies, are common in a family.

Atopic dermatitis
- Some people with the skin condition atopic dermatitis (eczema) also have a food allergy.[21]

Given the prevalence of peanuts in society, schools have taken initiative in safeguarding the environment for those individuals afflicted with life-threatening peanut allergies.[22] **Box 3** lists pitfalls to avoid when faced with severe peanut allergies.

Box 3
Pitfalls to avoid when faced with severe, life-threatening peanut allergies

1. Eating unlabeled foods

2. Accidental contamination of other foods (eg, jam, butter, or of eating utensils, food trays, table, and toys)

3. Unpackaged foods, such as buffet foods, free samples at grocery stores, and foods at pot luck dinner

4. Contamination during food preparation

5. Contamination during serving – using same utensil for a peanut and non–peanut-containing food

6. Trusting a nonpreparer of food to assert safety of the food (waiter, flight attendant, friend, etc.)

7. Trying a food to see if "still allergic" especially with an anaphylactic allergy.

8. Vending machines may have different foods at different times – thus, foods may be contaminated with traces of nuts if there were nuts in the dispensing machine before.

9. Nonfood sources of peanut, such as homemade playdough, homemade scented crayons, cosmetics or fishing lures with peanut, peanut shell stuffing in bean bags, draft stoppers, stuffed toys, peanut in animal food (eg, hamster, gerbil and bird food granules).

Adapted from FAQ about Food Allergies and District Food Guidelines. Forest Hills School District. Available at: http://www.foresthills.edu/userfiles/1522/FAQ%20about%20Food%20Allergies%20and%20District%20Food%20Guidelines.pdf. Accessed January 5, 2016.

Reducing the risk for anaphylaxis among peanut allergy sufferers is the ultimate goal. Recent advances in rendering the peanut itself less allergenic have been reported.[25]

Schools are the most common gathering place for children outside their respective homes. Food policies have evolved rapidly over the past decade to minimize exposure to the most common food allergens: peanuts, nuts, milk, and eggs.[26] Notices are now sent at the beginning of the school year reminding parents to not send nut-containing snacks or dairy products to school with their kids. Examples of such notices are listed in **Boxes 4** and **5**.[26] Replacing peanut oil at many schools with canola oil is now commonplace.[27]

Milk Allergies

The second most common food allergen, CMA, can develop in exclusively or partially breastfed infants, when cow milk protein is introduced into the feeding regime. The incidence of CMA is lower in exclusively breastfed infants compared with formula-fed or mixed-fed infants, and clinical reactions in the breastfed group are mostly mild to moderate. This might be related to lower levels of cow milk protein in breast milk compared with cow milk. Immunomodulators in breast milk and differences in gut flora between breastfed and formula-fed infants may also play a role.[28]

CMA results from an immunologic reaction to 1 or more milk proteins. Common offending milk proteins include whey and casein.[29] This immunologic basis distinguishes CMA from other adverse reactions to cow milk protein, such as lactose intolerance.[28]

Clinical reactions can be either immediate or delayed. Immediate reactions occur less than 2 hours after ingestion. The most frequent manifestations are immunoglobulin E (IgE)-mediated cutaneous (urticaria, angioedema, or acute flare-up of atopic eczema) and gastrointestinal (vomiting, diarrhea, or colic) reactions.[28] Anaphylaxis is a potential reaction and happens almost immediately (within minutes and up to 2 hours) after the ingestion of cow milk or dairy.[30]

Box 4
Milk and egg avoidance strategies

Anaphylactic reactions to milk and egg can occur when small quantities are ingested. Therefore, the allergic child must avoid all traces of milk/egg. Direction from Anaphylaxis Canada is that products containing milk and eggs are ones that are not to be banned or restricted, because trying to eliminate them is both unrealistic and a burden for the wider community.

Risk Reduction Strategies
Milk

It is imperative for teachers to collaborate with parents/guardians to establish suitable risk reduction strategies, along with following key safety rules, such as

- Carrying epinephrine autoinjector and not to eat without the autoinjector
- Wearing medical identification, such as a MedicAlert bracelet
- Eating only food items approved by parents/guardians
- Not trading or sharing foods, utensils, or food containers
- Washing hands before and after eating

Elementary schools have adopted different strategies to reduce the risk of exposure for milk and egg allergic children.

Milk products

Where milk products are allowed in classrooms, the following practices are implemented to reduce the risk:

- Children are given straws to put in bevel-topped milk containers (which are distributed through milk programs) and are taught to close the top once the straw is inserted.
- Children who bring milk from home are asked to bring it in a plastic bottle with a straw.
- Children at risk for milk allergy sit at a table where spillable milk products are not being consumed. Alternatively, they sit at the same table but not directly beside classmates who have spillable milk products (eg, milk and yogurt).
- Some parents of milk allergic children either take their child home for lunch on pizza days (where they have this option); others send their child with a homemade milk-free pizza or an alternative snack so they can still participate. Special care should be taken to ensure that children properly wash their hands after pizza lunches.

Risk Reduction Strategies: Egg

It is imperative for teachers to collaborate with parents/guardians to establish suitable risk reduction strategies.

Some food products that may contain egg protein are bread bushed with egg white; deli meats with egg; drinks, such as orange julep; and egg substitutes. Nonfood items that may contain egg protein include egg tempera paints, cosmetics, and shampoo.

In classrooms where there are egg-allergic children, parents and staff have worked to reduce the risk of accidental exposure by

- Avoiding egg in cooking classes or egg shells in craft activities (these includes both egg whites and yolks, either cooked or raw).
- Selecting activities that do not involve the use of egg for special activities (eg, Easter egg decorating or hunts [with real eggs]).
- Seating children with egg allergy away from those who bring eggs for lunch or snack (eg, hard boiled and egg salad sandwiches) or whose food may contain eggs (eg, mayonnaise).

Adapted from Canadian Society of Allergy and Clinical Immunology. Anaphylaxis in schools & other settings, 3rd edition. Available at: http://www.aaia.ca/en/Anaphylaxis_3rd_Edition.pdf.

Box 5
Peanuts and tree nuts avoidance strategies

Background

- Peanut allergy requires stringent avoidance and management plans, because it is one of the most common food allergies in children, adolescents, and adults.
- Reactions to peanuts are often more severe than to other foods.
- Peanut has been a leading cause of severe, life-threatening, and even fatal allergic reactions.
- Minute quantities of peanut, when ingested, can result in a life-threatening reaction.
- Cross-contamination is more likely to occur with peanut butter due to the adhesive nature of the peanut protein to other foods/surfaces.

For any of the signs and/or symptoms observed with an anaphylactic child, the first response is to follow the anaphylaxis emergency treatment plan, ACT:

- Administer the epinephrine autoinjector.
- Call 911, stating there is a child with anaphylaxis.
- Transport to hospital in an ambulance.

Sample strategies to reduce the risk of exposure to peanuts and tree nuts in the classroom and common school areas

- Communication (by letter, newsletter, school Web site, and so forth) is sent to each family in the school outlining that the school has students with life-threatening allergies to peanuts/tree nuts and requesting parent/guardian support in making the school a minimized allergen environment by not sending or bringing food products that contain or may contain peanuts and/or tree nuts.
- Include reminder items during holiday times and celebrations that the school is a minimized allergen environment and food items with peanut/tree nuts should not be brought on school site.
- Provide parents of students in an allergic child's class with information about how they can assist in supporting a safe learning environment. This communication should come directly from the school administration, not from parents of the allergic child.
- Inform parents that food items should not contain traces of peanuts/nuts for celebrations (eg, birthdays).
- Stress with staff to be vigilant in not having food items with peanuts and other nuts in the school and not to bring food products that may contain the allergen (eg, baked goods, such as donuts or cookies from doughnut shops) to staff meetings/lunches or special occasions (eg, birthdays).
- School fundraisers should avoid products containing the allergens (eg, peanuts and tree nuts) that the school is trying to minimize (eg, chocolate almonds).
- Teachers, particularly in the primary grades, should be aware of the possible peanut/nut allergens present in curricular materials
  - Playdough
  - Bean bags and stuffed toys (peanut shells are sometimes used)
  - Counting aids (beans and peas)
  - Science projects
  - Special seasonal activities
- Students with anaphylaxis should not be involved in garbage disposal, yard clean-ups, or other activities that could bring them into contact with food wrappers, containers, or debris.
- Foods are often stored in lockers and desks. Allowing anaphylactic students to keep the same desk all year may help prevent accidental contamination.

List of peanut/tree nut–free items

Recommendations are NOT to provide a list of "safe" peanut/tree nut–free snacks and so forth. The contents of products and the lines on which they are produced change often and cannot always guarantee that their product is peanut/tree nut–free. The best advice is to request the parents/caregivers read the contents of the packages and where it says, "may contain: nut products" – please do NOT send.

Adapted from Canadian Society of Allergy and Clinical Immunology. Anaphylaxis in schools & other settings, 3rd edition. Available at: http://www.aaia.ca/en/Anaphylaxis_3rd_Edition.pdf.

Delayed reactions are immunologic, non–IgE-mediated reactions and occur several hours, even days, after milk consumption. Skin and gastrointestinal manifestations are most commonly observed, typically inducing flare-ups of eczema or conditions, known as food protein–induced enterocolitis, enteropathy, and proctolitis.[30]

Diagnostic testing for milk allergies is discussed in detail elsewhere.[29] Skin prick testing (SPT) and radioallergosorbent test (RAST) (blood test used to determine the substances a subject is allergic to) are typical diagnostic standards of care. A summary of the recommendations for diagnostic testing is as follows:

- A formal challenge with cow milk remains the best diagnostic test.
- Food challenge should be performed with physician supervision regardless of food-specific IgE value.
- In settings where oral food challenge is not considered a requirement for making a diagnosis of IgE-mediated complementary and alternative medicine, a positive SPT and/or RAST can be used as diagnostic tests in cases of high pretest probability.
- In such settings, a negative SPT and/or RAST with whole milk can be used as rule-out tests in case of low pretest probability.
- In any case of high uncertainty, food challenges remain necessary.[28,29]

DIAGNOSIS

Diagnosis is typically based on clinical presentation (symptoms are discussed previously) and/or further allergen testing.

Food Allergen Challenge Test

For all individuals with suspected food allergies, a food allergen challenge test is usually recommended (**Fig. 2**).

Allergists typically administer this test in an office or, more rarely, in a hospital's intensive care setting. The procedure involves having the patient ingest a food item that has the presumed allergenic food substance within.

Double-blind, placebo-controlled testing is best undertaken to eliminate bias, such that the patient and physician are unaware of which food item contains the offending food allergen.[31] Reactions, if any, are documented and measured. If this initial test is negative for any reaction, an open challenge test can be administered where the patient knowingly ingests a food substance thought to induce allergic reactions. Should this test prove negative as well, the patient is not deemed allergic and is encouraged to consume age-appropriate amounts of the food substance on a regular basis.

Precautionary measures include advising individuals to carry an epinephrine auto-injector (EpiPen) for several months after having established a negative allergy test as a backup for unexpected reactions.[32]

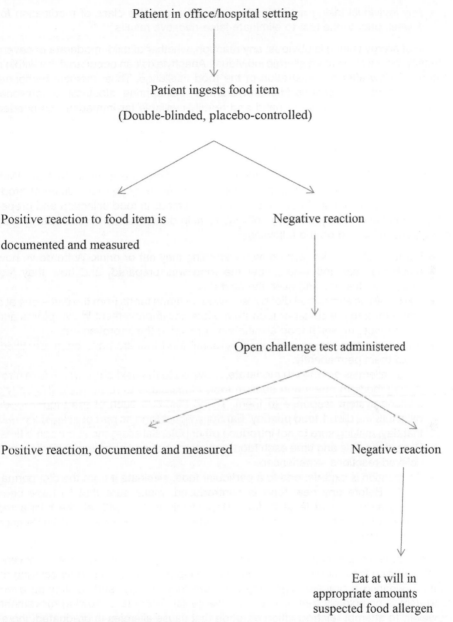

Fig. 2. Food allergen challenge test.

This type of allergy testing is not suitable for all allergic individuals. The following types of patients are not good allergy testing candidates:

- Patients with known or suspected multiple food or other allergies might develop a reaction to 1 or more food substances but there is no way to decipher which food substance generated the reaction.
- Asthma patients are deemed high risk, because allergic-type reactions might exacerbate underlying asthma and cause severe wheezing.

- Any individual taking antihistamines should cease this class of medication for 1 week prior to the test to eliminate false-negative results.[31,32]

Risk of allergy testing is obvious: any reaction, whether of mild, moderate or severe intensity, poses a risk to an allergic individual. Anaphylaxis can occur anytime within a 2-hour window after administration of the food challenge. Thus, medical personnel and appropriate medications (diphenhydramine, epinephrine, albuterol, prednisone, or prednisolone) should be on hand and readily available for immediate as-needed administration.[31,32]

TREATMENT OF FOOD ALLERGIES

Identification of a particular food allergy can sometimes be a tiresome task. With wheat, eggs, nuts, dairy, and so forth being components of so many different products, it is imperative to instruct patients to be fastidious in food selection and preparation and also in food journaling. Initially, to help determine what food allergy may exist, patients should do the following:

- For at least 2 weeks, write down everything they eat or drink. Write down how much they eat and when, how the food was prepared, and how they feel throughout the day and even the next day.
- Next, start an elimination diet by removing common foods from the diet—one at a time—for 2 to 6 weeks per food item. Note any improvement in symptoms and make a note of which food eliminations preceded the improvements.
- If food allergies are severe, once personal food triggers have been identified, avoid them permanently.
- If food allergies are mild to moderate, move on to the next step, which is reintroducing foods to retest and confirm food triggers and to re-evaluate the body's immune system response to them. To do this, add each of the trigger foods back into the diet, 1 food per day. Eat the suspect food as part of at least 2 meals that day, making sure to not introduce other potential allergens at the same time. Record the date and time each food is reintroduced and note any immediate and delayed reactions experienced.
- If a reaction is experienced to a particular food, eliminate it from the diet permanently. Before any new food is reintroduced, make sure that to have been symptom-free for at least 2 days. Repeat this testing with all the suspected trigger foods until figuring out exactly which ones cause the food intolerance or food allergy symptoms.[33]

Not all patients can reintroduce the offending food allergen into their diet. A severe, life-threatening food allergy requires life-preserving precautions, such as carrying an EpiPen, wearing a bracelet signifying a severe food allergy, and confirming every food item is completely free of the food allergen(s). There is a growing movement, however, to attempt reintroduction of foods that cause allergies in graduated, incrementally tiny doses. Dr Kari Nadeau, an allergist-immunologist at Stanford University, has attempted this process with ongoing successes.[34] This process is known as food oral immunotherapy and is being studied as a way to help treat food allergies. Under close supervision, a person takes in small daily doses of a food allergen by mouth or under the tongue. The goal is to try to make the immune system tolerate the allergen so that the body does not react as badly to it. This is called desensitization (discussed later). Now the paradigm of avoidance of specific, common food allergens in infancy, such as nuts, is being reversed, with exposure to peanuts and nut products in infancy considered a good thing among allergists.[35]

Strategies Designed to Alter the Immune Response to Food Allergens

Oral immunotherapy (discussed previously) is the most studied approach to modulating the immune system response to specific food allergens.[36] This approach has been discussed in detail elsewhere.[36] Increased amounts of the particular food allergen(s) are given in rapid fashion over a short course, followed by escalation of doses within a 2-week time frame, with the maintenance phase lasting up to several months to years.[36]

Clinical desensitization is the confirmation of the body's immune system responding less allergically to particular food allergen(s). Reduction in mast cell activity, basophil activation, and helper T cells along with changes in immunoglobulin profiles have been demonstrated.[36]

Scientific trials are being undertaken regarding how best to prevent food allergies.

The Enquiring About Tolerance study aims to find out how to best prevent food allergy in young children.[29] The study aims to find out whether introducing certain foods early in a child's diet along with continued breastfeeding could stop infants developing food allergy.[37] In this double-blind, placebo-controlled study, 1302 children were enrolled, split into 2 groups: 1 group received allergenic foods as of age 3 months onward, along with breast milk; the other group received breast milk exclusively until age 6 months. Children were then monitored until age 3 years and the rate of food allergies monitored and compared. Results are pending.[37]

Science has already confirmed that desensitization can occur for peanuts, milk, and eggs.[38–40]

Functional tolerance to food allergens has also been clinically proved, such that after the appropriate desensitization period patients are able to consume certain amounts of food allergens on an ad hoc basis without generating an allergic-type reaction.[41]

REFERENCES

1. Sicherer SH, Sampson HA. Food allergy: epidemiology, pathogenesis, diagnosis, and treatment. J Allergy Clin Immunol 2014;133(2):291–307.
2. Soller L, Ben Shoshan M, Harrington DW, et al. Overall prevalence of self-reported food allergy in Canada. J Allergy Clin Immunol 2012;130:986–8.
3. Jackson KD, Howie LD, Akinbami LJ. Trends in allergic conditions among children: United States 1997-2011. NCHS Data Brief 2013;(121):1–8.
4. Gupta R, Springston EE, Warrier MR, et al. The prevalence, severity and distribution of childhood food allergy in the United States. Pediatrics 2011;128(1):e9–17.
5. Boyce JA, Assa'ad A, Burks AW, et al. Guidelines for the diagnosis and management of food allergy in the United States: report of the NIAID-sponsored expert panel. J Allergy Clin Immunol 2010;126(Suppl):S1–58.
6. Decker WW, Campbell RL, Manivannan V, et al. The etiology and incidence of anaphylaxis in Rochester, Minnesota: a report from the Rochester Epidemiology Project. J Allergy Clin Immunol 2008;122(6):1161–5.
7. Available at: http://www.webmd.com/allergies/foods-allergy-intolerance. Accessed January 5, 2016.
8. Liu AH, Jaramillo R, Sicherer SH, et al. National prevalence and risk factors for food allergy and relationship to asthma: results from the National Health and Nutrition Examination Survey 2005-2006. J Allergy Clin Immunol 2010;126: 798–806.
9. Visness CM, London SJ, Daniels JL, et al. Association of obesity with IgE levels and allergy symptoms in children and adolescents: results from the National

Health and Nutrition Examination Survey 2005-2006. J Allergy Clin Immunol 2009; 123:1163–9.

10. Lack G. Update on risk factors for food allergy. J Allergy Clin Immunol 2012;129: 1187–97.

11. Untersmayr E, Jensen-Jarolim E. The role of protein digestibility and antacids on food allergy outcomes. J Allergy Clin Immunol 2008;121:1301–8.

12. Osborne NJ, Ukoumunne OC, Wake M, et al. Prevalence of eczema and food allergy is associated with latitude in Australia. J Allergy Clin Immunol 2012;129:865–7.

13. Vassallo MF, Banerji A, Rudders SA, et al. Season of birth and food allergy in children. Ann Allergy Asthma Immunol 2010;104:307–13.

14. Sheehan WJ, Graham D, Ma L, et al. Higher incidence of pediatric anaphylaxis in northern areas of the United States. J Allergy Clin Immunol 2009;124:850–2.

15. Available at: http://www.cdc.gov/healthyschools/foodallergies/index.htm. Accessed January 5, 2016.

16. Centers for Disease Control and Prevention. Voluntary guidelines for managing food allergies in schools and early care and education programs. Washington, DC: US Department of Health and Human Services; 2013.

17. Thygarajan A, Burks AW. American Academy of Pediatrics recommendations on the effects of early nutritional interventions on the development of atopic disease. Curr Opin Pediatr 2008;20(6):698–702.

18. Available at: http://www.fda.gov/downloads/Food/ResourcesForYou/Consumers/UCM220117.pdf. Accessed January 5, 2016.

19. Available at: http://acaai.org/allergies/types/food-allergies. Accessed January 5, 2016.

20. Savage JH, Kaeding AJ, Matsui EC, et al. The natural history of soy allergy. J Allergy Clin Immunol 2010;125:683–6.

21. Zhao X, Yang W, Chung S, et al. Reduction of IgE immunoreactivity of whole peanut (Arachis hypogaea L.) after pulsed light illumination. Food Bioprocess Technol 2014;7:2637–45.

22. FAQ about Food Allergies and District Food Guidelines. Forest Hills School District. Available at: http://www.foresthills.edu/userfiles/1522/FAQ%20about%20Food%20Allergies%20and%20District%20Food%20Guidelines.pdf. Accessed January 5, 2016.

23. Greer FR, Sicherer SH, Burks AW. Effects of early nutritional interventions on the development of atopic disease in infants and children: the role of maternal dietary restriction, breastfeeding, timing of introduction of complementary foods, and hydrolyzed formulas. Pediatrics 2008;121:183–91.

24. Available at: http://www.foodallergy.org/managing-food-allergies/at-camp. Accessed January 5, 2016.

25. Chang TT, Huang CC, Hsu CH. Inhibition of mite-induced immunoglobulin E synthesis, airway inflammation, and hyperreactivity by herbal medicine STA-1. Immunopharmacol Immunotoxicol 2006;28(4):683–95.

26. Goldenberg E. The best school policy for allergy and anaphylaxis management. Onespot Allergy. Available at: http://blog.onespotallergy.com/2011/03/the-best-school-policy-for-allergy-and-anaphylaxis-management/. Accessed January 5, 2016.

27. Available at: http://www.peanutallergy.com/articles/peanut-allergy/how-to-replace-peanut-oil-with-canola-oil. Accessed January 5, 2016.

28. Available at: http://www.worldallergy.org/professional/allergic_diseases_center/cows_milk_allergy_in_children/. Accessed January 5, 2016.

29. Fiocchi A, Brozek J, Schüneman H, et al. World Allergy Organization (WAO) Diagnosis and Rationale for Action against Cow's Milk Allergy (DRACMA) Guidelines. World Allergy Organ J 2010;3(4):57–161.
30. Simons FE, Ardusso LR, Bilò MB, et al. World Allergy Organization Guidelines for the Assessment and Management of Anaphylaxis. World Allergy Organ J 2011;4: 13–37.
31. Available at: http://my.clevelandclinic.org/health/diagnostics/hic-allergy-tests/hic-food-challenge-test. Accessed January 5, 2016.
32. Available at: http://www.anaphylaxis.org.uk/what-is-anaphylaxis/knowledgebase/food-challenges-as-a-way-of-testing-for-food-allergies. Accessed January 5, 2016.
33. Available at: http://www.drdavidwilliams.com/food-allergies-natural-treatments/. Accessed January 5, 2016.
34. Available at: http://www.nytimes.com/2013/03/10/magazine/can-a-radical-new-treatment-save-children-with-severe-allergies.html?_r=0. Accessed January 5, 2016.
35. Du Toit G, Robert G, Sayre PH, et al. Randomized trial of peanut consumption in infants at risk of peanut allergy. N Engl J Med 2015;372:803–13.
36. Adkinson NF Jr, Bochner BS, Burks W, et al. 8th edition. Middleton's allergy: principles and practice, vol. 1, 2014. p. 1374–7.
37. Available at: http://www.eatstudy.co.uk/. Accessed January 5, 2016.
38. Hsu CH, Lu CM, Chang TT. Efficacy and safety of modified Mai-Men-Dong-Tang for treatment of allergic asthma. Pediatr Allergy Immunol 2005;16(1):76–81.
39. Li XM, Brown L. Efficacy and mechanisms of action of traditional Chinese medicines for treating asthma and allergy. J Allergy Clin Immunol 2009;123(2): 297–306.
40. Netting M, Makrides M, Gold M, et al. Heated allergens and induction of tolerance in food allergic children. Nutrients 2013;5(6):2028–46.
41. Available at: http://www.mayoclinic.org/diseases-conditions/peanut-allergy/basics/symptoms/con-20027898. Accessed January 5, 2016.

Drug Allergy

Abdul Waheed, MD*, Tiffany Hill, MD, Nidhi Dhawan, MD

KEYWORDS

- Drug reaction • Drug allergy • Hypersensitivity • Presentation • Diagnosis
- Treatment • Prevention

KEY POINTS

- Adverse drug reactions can be classified as type A reactions and type B reactions. Type A reactions are defined as predictable, common, dose-dependent effects that are related to the pharmacologic actions of a drug.
- Drug allergy is considered a type B reaction and includes a range of immunologically mediated hypersensitivity reactions with different mechanisms and clinical presentations.
- Drug allergies are unpredictable in presentation and can present as mild as a maculopapular rash or as severe reactions, such as toxic epidermal necrosis or anaphylaxis.
- The diagnosis of drug allergy is made with careful history, physical examination, and sometimes allergy testing.
- A first step in the treatment of a drug allergy is to stop the offending agent. Mild drug allergies can be treated with first-generation antihistamines and topical/systemic steroids, but more severe reactions may require epinephrine and airway management.

INTRODUCTION/EPIDEMIOLOGY

All drugs have the possibility of causing side effects. These side effects are often labeled as "adverse drug reactions." Adverse drug reactions are common in both the inpatient and outpatient settings. They are between the fourth and sixth leading cause of death and attribute to more than 100,000 deaths in the United States.[1]

Adverse reactions can further be further categorized as type A reactions and type B reactions. Type A reactions are defined as predictable, common, dose-dependent effects that are related to the pharmacologic actions of a drug. Type B reactions are unpredictable, uncommon, not dose dependent, and are usually not related to the pharmacologic action of the drug.[2] Classic examples of type A reactions include bradycardia with propranolol or gastrointestinal bleed with nonsteroidal anti-inflammatory drugs. Approximately 80% of type A reactions fall into this

Disclosures: None.
Department of Family & Community Medicine, Milton S. Hershey Medical Center, Penn State College of Medicine, Hershey, PA, USA
* Corresponding author. Department of Family & Community Medicine, Milton S. Hershey Medical Center, Penn State College of Medicine, 845 Fishburn Road, Hershey, PA 17033.
E-mail address: awaheed1@hmc.psu.edu

Prim Care Clin Office Pract 43 (2016) 393–400
http://dx.doi.org/10.1016/j.pop.2016.04.005
0095-4543/16/$ – see front matter © 2016 Elsevier Inc. All rights reserved.

category.[3] Type B reactions, however, are immune-mediated or allergic-type reactions. These can present with manifestations as mild as a maculopapular rash to a more severe skin reaction such as toxic epidermal necrosis or even life-threatening syndromes like anaphylaxis.

Drug allergy or drug hypersensitivity is considered a Type B reaction, is unpredictable, and includes a range of immunologically mediated hypersensitivity reactions with different mechanisms and clinical presentations.[4]

RISK FACTORS

Drug allergy is a product of interplay of unique factors related to a patient and a drug.[4] Female individuals are more likely than male individuals to have drug allergies. In the Alergologica 2005 study, the female/male ratio for first-time consults for drug allergy was approximately 2:1. The incidence of self-reported drug allergy was also generally higher in female than in male individuals. Individuals with other disease states, such as human immunodeficiency virus (HIV) or herpes simplex virus are more likely to have drug allergies. Topical, intramuscular, or intravenous routes of drug administration are considered higher risk than oral formulations. Also, individuals receiving drugs for an extended period of time or multiple doses are at higher risk of developing drug allergy than those who receive a single large dose (**Table 1**).[5]

BASIC PATHOPHYSIOLOGY

As mentioned, adverse drug reactions are often incorrectly categorized and documented as a drug allergy. True drug allergies are immune-mediated reactions and should be distinguished from the many other types of reactions. As mentioned previously, there are 2 main categories of adverse drug reactions: type A and type B (**Fig. 1**). Most drug reactions are type A, with only approximately 20% or less classified as type B reactions.[3]

Type A is a drug reaction that is predictable and related to the pharmacodynamics of the drug.

Type B is divided into 4 groups with 1 type of immune-mediated group and 3 types of nonimmune reactions.

Table 1	
Common risk factors associated with drug allergy	
Patient Related	**Drug Related**
Viruses: human immunodeficiency virus, herpes simplex virus[2,7]	Route of administration[7]
Female gender[2,7]	Dose related[7]
Age[7]	High molecular weight[7]
Renal disease[2]	Hapten-forming drugs, such as penicillin and sulfamethoxazole[7]
Systemic lupus erythematosus[2]	—
Previous exposure[7]	—
Genetics (leading to idiosyncrasy)	—

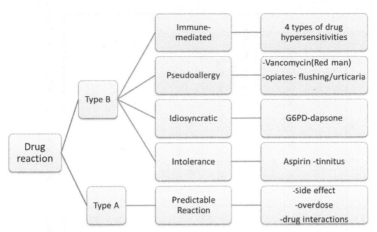

Fig. 1. Adverse drug reaction classification.

1. *Immune mediated:* 4 types of drug hypersensitivity based on Gell and Coomb's classification
2. *Intolerance:* a drug reaction that is not dose dependent
3. *Idiosyncrasy:* drug reaction due to genetic component
4. *Pseudoallergy:* a reaction that mimics an immune-mediated response by stimulating immune cells such as mast cells or immunoglobulin (Ig)E. This group also contains anaphylactoid reactions that mimic IgE-mediated anaphylaxis reaction. Despite the difference in mechanism, they should be treated the same.[6]

A classic example of pseudo allergy is aspirin-exacerbated respiratory disease. In patients who have preexisting asthma, bronchospasm may occur after consuming aspirin. Cyclo-oxygenase-1 inhibitors also may cause immune-mediated responses.[7]

MECHANISMS OF DRUG HYPERSENSITIVITY REACTIONS

Gell and Coombs suggested 4 basic types of immune-mediated drug hypersensitivity. Each type is classified into immediate or delayed response. Immediate reaction is defined as occurring within 1 hour, whereas delayed reaction may present 6 hours to weeks after exposure. Classifications of groups are also based on immune response, for example, IgE or T-cell mediated. Four types of hypersensitivity are summarized in **Table 2**.

IgE reactions typically occur after at least 1 exposure to medication. New developments show that an immediate response may even occur on first exposure and that antibodies may form during exposure to a different substance.[8]

As indicated previously, some drugs can present in several different types; antibiotics and heparin are classic examples. Heparin can present in all types, but type 1 is less common. Delayed reactions include heparin-induced thrombocytopenia, skin necrosis, and rashes.[9] Additionally, hypersensitivity reaction can be triggered by viruses. This usually occurs with delayed cell-mediated response as T cells are activated. The classic example of this occurs with administration of amoxicillin in the setting of Epstein-Barr virus mononucleosis producing a maculopapular reaction, but this also seen in patients with HIV who receive sulfonamides.

Table 2
Gell and Coombs 4 types of hypersensitivity

Clinical Presentation	Type I IgE-Mediated	Type II Cytotoxic	Type III Immune Complex	Type IV Delayed Cell Mediated
Onset	Immediate 30–60 min	Delayed	Delayed 1–3 wk	Delayed 48/72 h–wk
Immune response	Drug–IgE complex binds to mast cells causing release of inflammatory markers; in general, requires prior exposure to drug	Drug acts an antigen, binding to a cell. IgG/IgM coats the cell, targeting it for phagocytosis	Drug complexes deposits into various tissues	Involves T cell, which activates other effector cells (eosinophils, basophils, and monocytes)
Presentation	Urticaria, angioedema, anaphylaxis	Hemolytic anemia thrombocytopenia	Serum sickness Vasculitis Arthralgia Fever Arthus reaction	Contact dermatitis Steven Johnson DRESS TEN
Common offenders	Beta-lactam Neuromuscular blocking agent Quinolones Chemotherapy	Heparin –HIT type II Quinine/Quinidine NSAIDS Sulfonamides Carbamazepine	Penicillins Beta-lactam Sulfonamides Vaccines	Local anesthetics Dapsone

Abbreviations: DRESS, drug reaction with eosinophilia and systemic symptoms; HIT, heparin-induced thrombocytopenia; Ig, immunoglobulin; NSAID, nonsteroidal anti-inflammatory drug; TEN, toxic epidermal necrolysis.

CLINICAL PRESENTATION

The most common presentation of drug allergy is a maculopapular rash, which is commonly seen on the trunk and extremities (**Table 3**).[4] It is described as a flat, erythematous rash with small bumps. This type of rash can occur within days and up to 3 weeks.[4] Urticaria or hives is another common presentation of drug allergy and is described as a red, itchy, raised rash with or without edema and occurs within 1 hour of drug exposure.[10] Drug reaction with eosinophilia and systemic symptoms or better known as DRESS syndrome is diagnosed if at least 3 of the following criteria are met: skin rash; hematological abnormalities, such as eosinophilia or atypical lymphocytes in peripheral blood; abnormal liver enzymes; renal impairment; myocarditis; pneumonia.[10] More severe cutaneous manifestations of drug allergy include toxic epidermal necrosis (TEN) and Steven Johnson Syndrome (SJS). These severe presentations are rare and patients affected have high mortality rates. Patients will usually have vague symptoms, such as throat pain, fever, malaise, and stinging eyes.[10] Involvement of skin and mucous membranes usually occurs within a few days and initially presents on the face and trunk and eventually progresses to larger body areas. Erythematous macules, patches, flaccid blisters, and erosions are visible, and the spots have a gray to violet color.[10] A positive Nikolsky sign is sometimes present in individuals affected with SJS or TEN where gentle pressure at an uninvolved site leads to sloughing of the superficial skin.

DIAGNOSIS

Diagnosing drug allergy is difficult and can be challenging at times. Just like with any chief complaint, taking a thorough history is extremely important when trying to diagnose a drug allergy. A thorough history will help guide the clinician when ordering laboratory tests or diagnostic tests. It is important to know details such as when the rash erupted and how quickly; what medications the patient is on; were there any systemic symptoms; has this type of reaction occurred before; how long did the reaction last. The skin is the most common organ involved in drug allergies, so therefore a complete physical examination is necessary and crucial.

If one suspects an adverse drug reaction, there are further diagnostic tests that can be performed. For IgE-mediated or immediate drug reactions, skin prick testing and

Table 3 Common clinical presentations	
Classic Drug Reaction Pattern	**Clinical Presentation**
Generalized exanthema or maculopapular rash	Fine macules and papules; diffuse; most common presentation
Urticaria or "hives"	Raised lesions; well circumscribed; erythematous; pruritic; second most common presentation
Steven Johnson Syndrome	Flulike symptoms initially; followed by painful erythematous or purplish blisters; lip and facial swelling
TEN	Widespread erythema and necrosis; sloughing of skin; life threatening
DRESS	Cutaneous eruption; LAD; hepatic dysfunction; renal impairment; fever; eosinophilia

Abbreviations: DRESS, drug reaction with eosinophilia and systemic symptoms; LAD, lymphadenopathy; TEN, toxic epidermal necrolysis.

intradermal testing are commonly used and often times helpful. Beta-lactams are the most important drugs involved in immediate reactions and therefore skin prick testing is one diagnostic approach. Skin prick testing is performed by penetrating the skin with a lancet with the offending allergen, which elicits a localized reaction, whereas intradermal testing involves injecting the allergen into the dermis. Skin prick testing is usually done in 30 minutes and it is important to inform the patient to avoid antihistamines before skin prick testing so an appropriate immunologic response is mounted.

The most common in vitro technique to test for immediate drug reactions is serum-specific IgE assays. ImmunoCap is the most validated immunoassay and is widely used for evaluating immediate reactions to beta-lactams, mainly penicillins, with a specificity approaching 90% and a sensitivity of up to 50%.[7]

When skin prick testing or intradermal testing is negative, unavailable, or not validated, drug provocation test or graded challenges are the gold standard for identifying drugs that elicit an immediate reaction.[7]

For nonimmediate reactions, skin patch testing is more often used. This involves placing possible allergens at nonirritant concentrations on the patient's back for 48 hours under aluminum discs and then assessing for reactions.[4] These tests are not useful for the diagnosis of SJS or TEN.

TREATMENT

Treatment of both immune-mediated and pseudoallergy are based on clinical presentation. Mild reactions are considered to be subcutaneous, whereas moderate to severe reactions have a systemic effect. A thorough evaluation is imperative so as to triage appropriately (**Fig. 2**).

MANAGEMENT

Management heavily relies on proper establishment of the diagnosis (**Fig. 3**). Once a drug allergy is confirmed, the inciting drug should be avoided and alternative treatments may be used; but with inherent risk. Alternative treatments, however, are not without risk, and may produce a drug reaction due to cross reactivity (**Table 4**). This reactivity occurs with drugs that have similar structures.

Penicillin is the most common medication allergy. Up to 90% of patients with a history of penicillin allergy are able to tolerate penicillin.[11] Often, more expensive

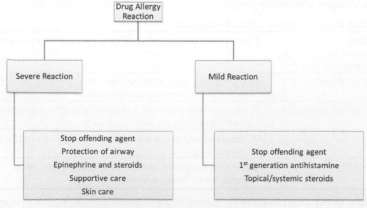

Fig. 2. Management strategies for drug allergy.

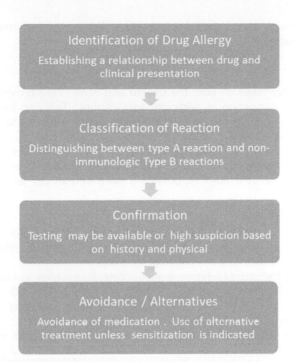

Fig. 3. Management algorithm.

antibiotics are used due to a reported "drug allergy." In particular, there is skin testing for the penicillin class available and it is recommended. In those patients who require treatment with penicillin, such as syphilis, desensitization can be performed. Desensitization is a process in which incremental doses of a drug are given to a patient

Table 4 Alternative medications that could be considered in allergic reactions	
Drug	**Alternative**
Penicillin	• Carbapenems and monopenems do not have a significant degree of cross reactivity. • Monopenems: Exception if there is a reaction to ceftazidime • Second and third-generation cephalosporins • First-generation cephalosporins
Cephalosporins	Higher degree of cross reactivity with first-generation cephalosporins and penicillin
Sulfonamides	• Any antibiotic • No cross reactivity with nonantibiotic sulfonamides • Exception sulfasalazine
Radiocontrast	May be used with pretreatment with steroids and antihistamine in nonsevere reactions
NSAIDs	Most reactions are caused by COX-1 inhibitors. COX-2 inhibitors are unlikely to have cross reactivity

Abbreviations: COX, cyclo-oxygenase; NSAID, nonsteroidal anti-inflammatory drug.
  Data from Warrington R, Silviu-Dan F. Drug allergy. Allergy Asthma Clin Immunol 2011;7(Suppl 1):S10; and Warrington R. Drug allergy causes and desensitization. Hum Vaccin Immunother 2012;8(10):1513–24.

to reduce the heightened sensitivity state and is usually performed in type 1, IgE-mediated reactions.[12]

PREVENTION

Prevention primarily relies on both the patient and health care providers playing an active role in the avoidance of particular medications. This can be done by first educating patients on drug allergy and risk. Next, clearly labeling the patient's chart with all known drug allergies and the severity of allergic syndrome is very important. Routine prescriptions of injectable epinephrine, such as EpiPen, are not recommended for all drug allergies. However, if patients have a moderate to severe allergic reaction or multiple allergy syndrome, providing them with an EpiPen may prevent an adverse outcome.

REFERENCES

1. Lazarou J, Pomeranz BH, Corey PN. Incidence of adverse drug reactions in hospitalized patients. JAMA 1998;279(15):1200–5.
2. Janet BC. Mechanisms of adverse drug reactions to biologics. In: Uetrecht J, editor. Adverse drug reactions. Toronto (Canada): Springer; 2010. p. 453.
3. Posadas SJ, Pichler WJ. Delayed drug hypersensitivity reactions–new concepts. Clin Exp Allergy 2007;37(7):989–99.
4. Warrington R, Silviu-Dan F. Drug allergy. Allergy Asthma Clin Immunol 2011; 7(Suppl 1):S10.
5. Thong BYH, Tan TC. Epidemiology and risk factors for drug allergy. Br J Clin Pharmacol 2011;71:684–700.
6. Baldo BA, Pham NH. Classification and descriptions of allergic reactions to drugs. In: Baldo BA, Phan NH, editors. Drug allergy: clinical aspects, diagnosis, mechanisms, structure-activity relationships. New York: Springer; 2013. p. 15.
7. Romano A, Torres MJ, Castellas M, et al. Diagnosis and management of drug hypersensitivity reactions. J Allergy Clin Immunol 2011;127(3 Suppl):S67–73.
8. Whearley LM, Plaut M, Schwaninger JM, et al. Reports from the National Institute of Allergy and Infectious Diseases workshop on drug allergy. J Allergy Clin Immunol 2015;136(2):262–71.
9. Bircher A, Harr T, Hohenstein L, et al. Hypersensitivity reactions to anticoagulant drugs: diagnosis and management options. Allergy 2006;61(12):1432–40.
10. Szegedi A, Remenyik E. Drug hypersensitivity reactions. In: Katsambas A, Lotti T, Dessinioti C, et al, editors. European handbook of dermatological treatments. Berlin; Heidelberg (Germany): Springer Verlag; 2015. p. 219–31.
11. Khan DA, Solensky R. Drug allergy. J Allergy Clin Immunol 2010;125(2):S126–37.
12. Celik GE, Pichler WJ, Adkinson NF. Drug allergy. In: Adkinson NF, Brochner BS, Busse WW, et al, editors. Allergy, principles and practice. 7th edition. Philadelphia: Elsevier; 2007. p. 1274–95.

Respiratory Allergic Disorders

Jason Raymond Woloski, MD[a],*, Skye Heston, MD[a],
Sheyla Pamela Escobedo Calderon, MD[b]

KEYWORDS

- Allergic • Asthma • Allergic bronchopulmonary aspergillosis
- Hypersensitivity pneumonitis

KEY POINTS

- Allergic asthma is a chronic, reversible, bronchoconstriction influenced by an allergic trigger.
- Allergic bronchopulmonary aspergillosis (ABPA) is a hypersensitivity reaction due to bronchi colonization by *Aspergillus* species.
- Hypersensitivity pneumonitis (HP) refers to lung inflammation from airborne environmental antigens, such as dust and mold.

ALLERGIC ASTHMA

Introduction

Asthma is described as a chronic, reversible, inflammatory disease, accompanied by airway hyper-responsiveness and bronchoconstriction.[1-3] Common symptoms include wheezing, dyspnea, chest tightness, and coughing.[1-3] The number of individuals afflicted with asthma continues to rise, with worldwide prevalence at approximately 300 million individuals.[1,4]

Asthma can be classified as allergic versus nonallergic types. Several different asthma triggers have been identified, including exercise, tobacco smoke, infections, cold air, and allergens.[2,3] Allergic asthma, previously referred to as extrinsic asthma, is the term used to describe the influence of allergens in the development of asthma.[5,6] Conversely, nonallergic asthma, formerly intrinsic asthma, should be considered when allergic etiology is ruled out after careful history, physical examination, and allergy testing.[6,7]

The authors have nothing to disclose.
[a] Department of Family Medicine, Penn State Hershey Medical Center, 500 University Drive, H154, PO Box 850, Hershey, PA 17033-0850, USA; [b] Peruvian Society of Family and Community Medicine, Ortega y Gasset 315, Calera, Surquillo, Lima, Peru
* Corresponding author.
E-mail address: jwoloski@hmc.psu.edu

Epidemiology/Pathophysiology

Allergic asthma patients tend to have earlier age of onset in comparison to nonallergic asthmatics (15.8 ± 1.3 vs 32.2 ± 2.3).[5] Boys and men are more prone to the allergic asthma subtype, whereas girls and women are more likely to have nonallergic asthma. One study concluded nonallergic asthma patients have a male-to-female ratio of 0.8 to 1.2.[5] Smoking status does not seem to differ between allergic versus nonallergic asthmatics.[5]

Both genetic and environmental factors play a role in the development of atopy and asthma, with several common gene loci identified among allergic asthmatics.[8] The presence of maternal asthma has been thought to play a role to a larger degree than paternal asthma.[9] One theory suggests that the combination of genetic suscep- tibility and in utero maternal exposures induces more of a type 2 helper T cell (Th2) im- munity response, thus increasing the risk of asthma from allergic sensitization early in life.[9,10] With infants spending more time indoors than outdoors, potential indoor aller- gens are also thought to lead to allergic sensitization and asthma in select high-risk children.[1] Early childhood exposure to domestic animals, however, has been shown to add a protective effect against the development of atopy and wheezing.[11]

Allergic asthma is initiated by the production of antigen-specific T cells to aller- gens.[12] The allergic asthma pathway is triggered on re-exposure of the allergen after the initial sensitization.[13] The term, *atopy*, refers to the immunoglobulin E (IgE) anti- body production to low doses of allergens.[5,6] In allergic asthma, allergens cross-link IgE on the surface of mast cells, resulting in the release of histamine, prostaglandins, and cytokines.[6,13,14] In turn, Th2 cell recruitment, increased mucus production, and bronchoconstriction are seen.[6,13,14] Cytokines that participate in the inflammatory response and the asthma pathway include interleukin (IL)-4, IL-13, IL-5, and IL-9.[6,10,15]

In patients with allergic asthma, acute infections often result in exacerbations of asthma. It has been suggested that respiratory syncytial virus bronchiolitis in infancy can give rise to asthma, with subsequent amplification of allergic inflammation.[16] Another example is the increased number of asthma exacerbations related to rhino- virus infection in patients with high IgE titers to allergens, such as dust mites.[17]

An overwhelming association with concurrent allergic rhinitis has been seen among individuals with allergic asthma, with allergic rhinitis commonly preceding the onset of asthma.[2,3,7,11,18] Allergic rhinitis serves as an independent risk factor for future devel- opment of asthma, due to the similar Th2 immune cell involvement, triggering mast cell and eosinophil involvement.[7,15] Allergic rhinitis may also lead to increased mouth breathing, thus increasing exposure of the lower respiratory system to allergens un- able to be filtered by the nose.[11] Comorbid asthma with allergic rhinitis has been linked to increased emergency room visits and asthma attacks in comparison to individuals with asthma alone.[7]

Repeated allergen exposure subsequently results in recurring inflammation of the lungs and bronchial hyper-reactivity.[3,17] Many different allergens have been cited as potential triggers for patients with allergic asthma, including dust mites, cockroach res- idue, furred animals, molds, and pollen.[2,3,19] Food allergy is not a common trigger for allergic asthma symptoms.[20] New investigations using mouse models are also analyzing the potential role of atrial natriuretic peptide on the respiratory system, partic- ularly involvement inducing a Th2 immune cell response during acute allergic asthma.[21]

Clinical Presentation/Diagnosis

On diagnosis of asthma, a clinician should attempt to differentiate between allergic and nonallergic asthma. Hay fever and seasonal exacerbations of asthma favor allergic etiology.[5] Older age, female gender, nasal polyps, and forced expiratory volume in the first second of expiration (FEV_1) below 80% favor nonallergic asthma, because allergic asthmatics have a higher baseline FEV_1.[5] One study also cited 38.3% of allergic asthmatics reported a history of allergic dermatitis.[5]

Nonallergic asthmatics have worsening of symptoms in the autumn and winter months, with fewer exacerbations in the summer compared with allergic asthmatics.[5] Seasonal exacerbations are still common with allergic asthmatics, correlating with the seasonal increases of the individual's sensitive allergen.[20]

A patient's age is an important factor when developing a differential diagnosis. Upper airway diseases, laryngotracheomalacia, vascular rings, laryngeal webs, vocal cord dysfunction, foreign body, viral bronchiolitis, cystic fibrosis, and bronchopulmonary dysplasia are all important considerations in infants and children.[3] Adults should be evaluated for chronic obstructive pulmonary disease, congestive heart failure, pulmonary embolism, mechanical obstruction from tumors, or drug-induced cough.[3]

Confirmation of allergen sensitivity can be performed using skin tests to usual aeroallergens.[5] The difficulty often arises that many allergen triggers are not easily identifiable to patients, such as dust mites, cockroaches, and fungi.[17]

Clinical clues to the diagnosis of asthma include episodic symptoms of airway hyper-responsiveness.[3] A thorough history and physical often identify symptoms of cough, wheezing, shortness of breath, and chest tightness.[2,3] Personal and family history of asthma, allergics, or eczema should be solicited to identify possible allergic component.[3,15] Patterns of symptoms, such as seasonal exacerbations, nocturnal awakenings, changes with weather, stress-induced symptoms, and exercise are also important diagnostic clues.[3] Similarly, environmental exposure history should be explored to identify potential precipitating factors. These include pets, smoke, mold, dust, and vapors in the home.[2,3] Individuals with comorbid allergic rhinitis, sinusitis, or bronchopulmonary dysplasia may also be at increased risk for developing asthma, in particular allergic asthma.[3]

Due to the reversibility of the asthmatic symptoms, physical examination may not identify any chest findings, wheezing, use of accessory muscles, or increased work of breathing between exacerbations. Clinicians should also be alert, however, for increased nasal secretions, mucosal swelling, and nasal polyps, along with skin findings, such as eczema or atopic dermatitis, which can support the diagnosis.[2,3]

Using spirometry, an increase in FEV_1 of greater than 200 mL and at least 12% from baseline measure should be seen after inhalation of short-acting β_2-agonist.[2,3] This suggests the reversibility of the airway obstruction.[2,3]

Management/Treatment

Regardless of the cause or phenotype of the asthma, management focuses on relieving bronchoconstriction and preventing exacerbations. A stepwise approach to asthma treatment involves long-term control with inhaled corticosteroids, long-acting β_2-agonists, and leukotriene modifiers.[2,3,6] Similarly, short-acting β_2-agonists, anticholinergics, and systemic corticosteroids can be used for acute symptoms.[2,3,6] Providing patients with a written asthma action plan for daily control and exacerbation management is also a vital component of the treatment plan.[3]

Reducing allergen exposure is another method for reduction of allergic asthma triggers and symptoms. This includes household activities, such as polishing floors and frequent washing of bedding in the home, to reduce mite exposure.[2,17] Patients with pollen allergies can be advised to keep windows closed, whereas individuals with pet allergies should inquire about prior pets living in the dwelling when moving into a new house or apartment.[2,17] Limiting time spent outdoors during peak pollen times is also beneficial.[2] If removal of a pet from the home is not an option, high-efficiency particulate air filters can be helpful.[2,19]

If a patient is at least 12 years of age with severe persistent allergic asthma (symptoms persisting despite inhaled corticosteroid), immunomodulation with omalizumab, an anti-IgE medication, can be considered as an add-on therapy.[2-4,6,16] Although historically omalizumab was recommended for patients 12 years of age and older, in 2013 the UK National Institute for Health and Care Excellence set 6 years of age as the minimal age.[4] Functioning as a monoclonal antibody, omalizumab works by binding to free IgE in the serum, inhibiting the binding of IgE to mast cell and basophil receptors.[3,4] Administration involves a subcutaneous injection every 2 to 4 weeks.[2] Omalizumab also provides an anti-inflammatory effect through the reduction of sputum and bronchial tissue eosinophilia.[16] A 2014 Cochrane review concluded when using omalizumab as an adjunctive therapy to inhaled steroids the drug was effective in decreasing the number of asthma exacerbations and hospitalizations and reducing patient doses of inhaled steroids.[4] The drug was found well tolerated overall but some injection site reactions have been reported.[4] The expense of omalizumab is a limit to its widespread use.[4]

Subcutaneous allergen immunotherapy can be considered for the suggested allergen as well.[2,3,6,22] This recommendation should be used with caution, however, because injection immunotherapy carries a risk of severe anaphylaxis.[2,22] A 2010 Cochrane review did show that injection immunotherapy reduces asthma symptoms and the use of asthma medications while improving bronchial hyper-reactivity.[22] Immunotherapy is more effective, however, in children than older patients.[23] Similarly, better results are seen when initiated early in the disease process.[23]

Comorbid allergic asthma with allergic rhinitis has a negative effect on asthma control.[7] Although data on the effects of treating allergic rhinitis on asthma control are conflicting, in general treatment of upper airway symptoms, such as rhinitis or sinusitis, has the potential to improve lower airway asthma symptoms.[3,7] Other methods of allergen control include dust mite mattress and pillow covers, routine washing of bedding, removing carpets and stuffed toys, frequent vacuuming, dehumidification of basements, and cleansing of mold.[2,3] Maintaining the humidity in the home below 50% has been shown to inhibit mite growth and reduce bronchial hyper-reactivity.[2,20]

There have also been several studies evaluating the effectiveness of complementary and alternative medicine practices for the prevention and treatment of asthma. These include yoga, herbals, and acupuncture.[24] Similarly, studies have been performed looking at the potential benefits of a diet rich in antioxidants and vitamin C in asthma prevention and treatment.[24]

In 2010, an update to the "Allergic Rhinitis and its Impact on Asthma (ARIA) guidelines" was published.[18] The update focused on recommendations focused on the primary, secondary, and tertiary prevention of allergy, allergic rhinitis, and asthma.[18] Recommendations included total avoidance of tobacco smoke, exclusive breast feeding for at the first 3 months of life, interventions to reduce the risk of developing dust mite exposure, minimization of occupational allergen exposures, and use of intranasal glucocorticosteroids for allergic rhinitis.[18] Moreover, for patients with allergic rhinitis and asthma, subcutaneous specific immunotherapy for the treatment of asthma, along with monoclonal antibody against IgE when symptoms progress despite treatment and allergen avoidance, is recommended.[18]

Future therapeutic strategies may involve medications that target allergen-derived peptides, along with the potential for creation of allergen vaccinations.[16] Treatment plans hopefully can be tailored to individual patients, keeping in mind environmental and genetic influences on a patient's asthma.[3] Other novel drug therapy targets include IL-5, IL-4, and IL-13, due to their role eosinophil production, recruitment, and proliferation as well as inflammation.[6,10] Several phase 2 and phase 3 drug studies are currently being conducted.[6,10] Studies in mouse models of allergic asthma are examining anti-inflammatory and decreased airway hyper-responsiveness properties of cyclic nitroxide radical therapies aimed at combating oxidative stress.[12]

ALLERGIC BRONCHOPULMONARY ASPERGILLOSIS
Introduction

ABPA is a complex hypersensitivity reaction, often in patients with asthma or cystic fibrosis (CF), which occurs when bronchi become colonized by *Aspergillus* species.[25–27]

ABPA has been described in patients with other chronic obstructive pulmonary diseases and in association with allergic fungal sinusitis, bronchocentric granulomatosis, hyper-IgE (Buckley) syndrome, and chronic granulomatous disease. In cases of these neutrophil disorders, differentiating between ABPA and an invasive disease related to *Aspergillus* is sometimes difficult.[28]

Epidemiology

This disease was first reported in 1890 and was later described in 1952 in 12 asthmatics with recurrent pulmonary infiltrates, eosinophilia (blood and sputum), and *Aspergillus hyphae* in their sputum.[29]

ABPA occurs primarily in patients with asthma (2%–32%) or with CF (1%–15%).[30–37] The Epidemiologic Registry of Cystic Fibrosis reported that ABPA prevalence was 7.8% in 2000 (ranging from 2.1% in Sweden to 13.6% in Belgium). The prevalence of ABPA was low in patients who were less than 6 years old.[38] When screening was performed in patients with persistent asthma, the prevalence was between 1% and 2%.[38,39]

Clinical Presentation

ABPA occurs in nonimmunocompromised patients, in the absence of invasive aspergillosis.[26] The clinical picture of ABPA is dominated by asthma complicated by recurrent episodes of bronchial obstruction, fever, malaise, expectoration of brownish mucus plugs, peripheral blood eosinophilia, and, at times, hemoptysis. Wheezing is not always evident, and some patients present with asymptomatic pulmonary consolidation.

Some patients who seem to have had no history of asthma or CF and then present with chest radiographic infiltrates and lobar collapse are found to have ABPA. Patients may have histories of intermittent mild asthma (exercise-induced bronchospasm) before their ABPA was diagnosed. Conversely, the asthma might have been persistent moderate or severe (corticosteroid dependent).[38,40]

Mold-allergic patients with asthma or ABPA experience acute respiratory symptoms of asthma or develop an episode of ABPA pulmonary eosinophilia after exposure to an especially moldy environment.[41]

The 5 stages proposed by Patterson and colleagues[41] remain useful. These stages are not phases of a disease, and in each case the physician should attempt to determine the stage that is present. The stages are presented in **Table 1**.[42]

A relationship between the level of exposure to *Aspergillus* and the occurrence of ABPA has not been clearly identified, although it has been suggested that high levels of exposure are associated with APBA exacerbations.[43]

Table 1
Stages of allergic bronchopulmonary aspergillosis

Stage	Description	Radiographic Infiltrates	Total Serum Immunoglobulin E
I	Acute	Upper lobes or middle lobe	Sharply elevated
II	Remission	No infiltrate and patient off prednisone for more 6 mo	Elevated or normal
III	Exacerbation	Upper lobes or middle lobe	Sharply elevated
IV	Corticosteroid-dependent asthma	Often without infiltrates, but intermittent infiltrates might occur	Elevated or normal
V	End stage	Fibrotic, bullous, or cavitary lesions	Might be normal

From Greenberger PA. Allergic bronchopulmonary aspergillosis. J Allergy Clin Immunol 2002;110: 687; with permission.

Radiographic Features

A chest radiograph may show parenchymal infiltrates (usually involving the upper lobes), atelectasis due to mucoid impaction, and several findings characteristic of bronchiectasis[43]:

- Tramline shadows due to thickened walls of nondilated bronchi
- Parallel lines due to the presence of ectatic bronchi
- Ring shadows due to mucus-filled bronchi or small abscesses seen next to pulmonary blood vessels
- Toothpaste shadows due to mucoid-impacted bronchi
- Gloved-finger shadows due to intrabronchial exudates with bronchial wall thickening
- Perihilar infiltrates may simulate hilar adenopathy

CT in patients with ABPA can have cylindrical, varicose, and cystic bronchiectasis that involves multiple bronchi. Thus, as seen on high-resolution CT, proximal bronchiectasis can be present in patients with asthma in the absence of ABPA; however, the CT results in patients with ABPA should have more areas of involvement.[44–46]

Pulmonary Testing

Most patients have airflow obstruction and air trapping with reduced FEV_1 and increased residual volume; a positive bronchodilator response is found in less than one-half of patients. Individuals with bronchiectasis or fibrosis may exhibit a mixed obstructive and restrictive pattern. A minority of patients have a reduction in diffusing capacity, an abnormality that may be more common in the presence of bronchiectasis.[47–55]

Diagnosis

Based on current recommendations, CF patients should be screened for ABPA each year from 6 years or in response to clinical suggestions of ABPA.[28] There is no individual test to establish a diagnosis of ABPA. The major reason for pursuing the diagnosis is that the condition responds to glucocorticoid therapy, and early detection and treatment may reduce the risk of progression to fibrotic disease. Diagnosis is usually confirmed by use of clinical, radiographic, and immunologic criteria.[25,29,30,47]

A skin prick test should be the first step in an asthmatic being evaluated for ABPA. A negative prick skin test followed by negative intradermal reactivity to *Aspergillus* virtually excludes ABPA from consideration.

If the prick test is positive, serum total IgE and precipitins to *Aspergillus* should be assayed. ABPA is excluded if the serum total IgE concentration is less than 417 IU/mL (1000 ng/mL) or if serum precipitins to *Aspergillus* are negative. IgE levels, like levels of blood eosinophilia, may decrease but generally do not normalize if a patient is receiving glucocorticoids. If the serum total IgE is greater than 417 IU/mL (>1000 ng/mL) and the precipitin test is positive for *Aspergillus*, then a presumptive diagnosis of ABPA is made. The presence of at least a 2-fold elevation in specific anti-*Aspergillus* IgE and IgG indices (compared with pooled serum of *Aspergillus*-sensitized non-ABPA asthmatics) indicates seropositive ABPA rather than sensitization to *Aspergillus* in asthmatics without ABPA.

Management/Treatment

The 2008 Infectious Diseases Society of America guidelines recommend that therapy for ABPA should consist of a combination of glucocorticoids and itraconazole.[56] The treatment is based on oral corticosteroids for 6 to 8 weeks at acute phase or exacerbation and itraconazole is now recommended and validated at a dose of 200 mg/d for a duration of 16 weeks. Children should receive 5 mg/kg per day given either once a day or, if the total dose exceeds 200 mg/d, in divided twice-daily doses with food. Liver function tests should be monitored monthly for any evidence of hepatotoxicity.[26,27,30,57]

The glucocorticoid dose varies with the stage of disease. Inhaled steroids may help control symptoms of asthma but do not have documented efficacy in preventing acute episodes of ABPA. An acute flare of ABPA (stage I) is treated with 0.5 mg/kg to 1.0 mg/kg of prednisone daily for 14 days, followed by conversion to an every-other-day regimen and a slow taper over 3 to 6 months.[58,59] The clinical response to glucocorticoids should be monitored with serial measurement of the serum total IgE concentration every 1 to 2 months.[57]

Itraconazole is thought to work by reducing the antigenic stimulus for bronchial inflammation.[56] The antifungal effects can be inferred by reduce specific *Aspergillus* IgG.[58] Another possible contributor to itraconazole action is by impairing metabolism of the glucocorticoid, thereby raising plasma levels.[59,60]

Successful use of voriconazole in ABPA has been reported in case reports and in a retrospective case series describing symptomatic, serologic, and radiographic features.[61–63] Whether voriconazole is superior to itraconazole in ABPA remains unknown, although voriconazole has distinct advantages to itraconazole, such as improved tolerance and bioavailability. The same case series suggests that the newer azole agent, posaconazole, may be effective for ABPA as well.[63]

A potential additional therapy that may be beneficial in the treatment of ABPA is omalizumab, a humanized monoclonal antibody against IgE. Proof of efficacy in ABPA for patients with and without CF awaits more definitive clinical trials.

Immunotherapy with fungal allergens has not been evaluated in high-quality studies. Evidence to support the initiation of fungal immunotherapy for the treatment of ABPA is lacking.[64]

HYPERSENSITIVITY PNEUMONITIS
Introduction

HP is a syndrome associated with lung inflammation from the inhalation of airborne antigens, such as molds and dust. HP has complex and diverse causes and is known by several different names, including extrinsic allergic alveolitis, farmer's lung, and pigeon breeder's disease, to name a few. Potential irritants are present in many different environments, ranging from different types of molds on hay, tobacco, and potatoes to coffee bean dust, tea plant debris, detergents, pesticides, and resins.[65]

Epidemiology

The prevalence and incidence are difficult to define and often under-reported, altogether mistaken for something else, and most of the data available are from studies done on farmers and bird handlers.[65,66] The most commonly known and seen throughout the United States is farmer's lung,[67] with an estimated prevalence of 9% of farmers in higher humidity zones and 2% in drier zones. Variation in the estimated prevalence in the United States alone is anywhere from 420 to 3000 affected per 100,000. The United Kingdom, France, and Finland have similarly varying ranges reported.[68,69] Bird owners' prevalence is even less known but estimates range from 20 to 20,000 per 100,000 in the United States.[70]

Incidence of HP is even harder to estimate given that it is often misdiagnosed because of the strong seasonality of symptoms, which gets it confused with seasonal allergies and viral upper respiratory infections. Cigarette smoke has been shown to decrease the rate of HP,[71,72] which has only compounded the confusion in the diagnosis because many high-risk populations may have a lower incidence than expected given their high levels of environmental exposure because of their tobacco use. Smoke exposure has been proposed to decrease the antibody response to inhaled irritants, which are proposed to cause HP.[73]

The highest-risk professions are vegetable and dairy farmers, those exposed to ventilation and humidified air, bird and poultry handlers, veterinarians and animal handlers, grain and processed food handlers, construction workers, and those exposed to processed wood, plastic, and other industrial chemicals.[74–78] Other high-risk groups that have been reported are office workers with high humidified or forced air, lifeguards, and automobile industrial workers exposed to polyurethane.[79–82]

Some of the suspected irritants are listed, but this is by no means an exhaustive list:

Farmer's lung: fungal spores, tobacco plant debris, coffee-bean dust, tea plant debris, grain dust (mixture of dust, silica, fungi, insects, and mites), and wood pulp debris

Water-related pneumonitis related to humidified air, hot tubs, or saunas

Thermoactinomyces (*T vulgaris*, *T sacchari*, and *T candidus*), *Klebsiella oxytoca*, *Cladosporium* sp, mycobacterium avium complex, and aerosolized endotoxin from pool-water sprays and fountains

Poultry/animal-related pneumonitis: droppings, feathers, chicken products, rat urine, dust/dandruff, bat droppings, fish meal, and oyster shells

Chemical exposures: diphenylmethane diisocyanate, sodium diazobenzene sulfate, copper sulfate (Bordeaux mixture), pyrethrum (pesticide), phthalic anhydride (heated epoxy resin), aerosolized metal working fluid, cotton mill dust, and tannic acid

Clinical Presentation

There has been an evolution in the classification and diagnosis of HP. The original classification was simply acute, subacute, and chronic. In 1982, the Boyd classification was proposed for acute progressive, acute intermittent nonprogressive, and nonacute subtypes. In 1996, the Cormier classification divided it into active and residual, and finally in 2011 the Selma classification proposed was active nonprogressive and intermittent, acute progressive and intermittent, and chronic nonprogressive and progressive.[83] This article uses the original classification for simplicity and because none of the other classifications have been as widely accepted.

Classification

Acute HP is by far the most common and easier to distinguish because there is often heavy exposure to an inciting agent in a patient's recent history. Patients often present with rapid onset of fevers chills malaise, nausea, cough, chest tightness, dyspnea without wheezing, tachypnea, and diffuse fine crackle.[84] Removal from irritant can result in resolution in symptoms as quickly as 12 hours or as long as several days to even several weeks. The disease may reoccur with re-exposure, but data are lacking to show if severity of symptoms are accelerated or minimized with repeat exposures and it likely depends on the environmental irritant.

Subacute represents a more gradual development of symptoms and is represented by gradual development of productive cough, dyspnea, fatigue, anorexia, and weight loss.[85] Symptoms are often persistent for several days to weeks and often do not resolve as spontaneously after removal of irritant as they do in an acute presentation.[86] In some but not all studies, there is a better overall prognosis in acute versus subacute presentations and chronic exposure and disease presentations.[87]

Clinical presentation in chronic HP may lack an obvious history of acute irritant exposure and a symptomatic episode and patients usually report an insidious onset of cough, dyspnea, fatigue, and weight loss. Digital clubbing may be seen in advanced disease and may help predict clinical deterioration. Symptoms correlating to pulmonary fibrosis are distinguishing symptoms and may correlate with increased mortality.[88] Because the initial exposure may be difficult to identify, many patients suffering with chronic HP may have been misdiagnosed with idiopathic pulmonary fibrosis because they can be difficult to distinguish clinically.[89] Removal from exposure usually results in only partial improvement.

Diagnosis

A comprehensive history with a well-identified exposure to an irritant known to cause HP in patients with clinical and radiologic features consistent with HP should lead to a strong clinical suspicion of HP. There is no single pathognomonic clinical presentation of HP. Simple avoidance of a suspected agent and subsequent resolution of symptoms can be significant in the diagnosis. A careful environmental history is essential, and at times physicians may choose to have a patient's environment inspected by an experienced industrial hygienist. Occasionally, other diagnostic procedures are required. Diagnosis is likely if pulmonary function tests may indicate an interstitial lung disease; chest imaging is consistent with ground-glass opacities, centrilobular nodules, fibrosis, emphysema, or more frequently a combination of these; and there are antibodies to the suspected antigen. Bronchoalveolar lavage has been used to the diagnosis but is not necessary and biopsies are rarely needed. Provocation tests are not necessary for the diagnosis and belong more in research procedures. There have been proposed diagnostic criteria but they have not had any recent consensus agreements nor been recently updated, the most recent diagnostic criteria proposed in 1996.[90–93]

Diagnostic Criteria

1. Identified contact to insulting antigen(s) recognized by (A) history of exposure, (B) investigations of the environment that confirm the presence of an inciting antigen,[94] or (C) positive specific IgG antibodies in serum against the identified antigen (serum

precipitins). A positive precipitin test even in the presence of a clear history of exposure to the identified antigen is merely suggestive of, rather than diagnostic of, a potential cause.

2. Compatible clinical, radiographic, or physiologic findings: (A) respiratory symptoms and signs like shortness of breath, wheezing, crackles, cough, weight loss, febrile episodes, and fatigue, if symptoms (as discussed previously) present shortly after suspected exposure than they become even more significant in the diagnosis; (B) reticular, nodular, or ground-glass opacity on chest imaging; (C) altered spirometry and/or lung volumes (may be restrictive, obstructive, or mixed pattern), reduced diffusing capacity lung for carbon monoxide, altered gas exchange either at rest or with exercise testing.

3. Bronchoalveolar lavage with lymphocytosis: (A) usually with low CD4-to-CD8 ratio, (B) positive specific immune response to the antigen by lymphocyte transformation testing (currently not available in most centers)

4. Positive inhalation challenge testing by (A) re-exposure to the environment, (B) inhalation challenge to the suspected antigen in a hospital setting

5. Histopathology showing compatible changes: (A) poorly formed, noncaseating granulomas or (B) mononuclear cell infiltrate

Definite hypersensitivity pneumonitis

A patient is considered to have definite HP under the following circumstances:

Criteria 1, 2, and 3 are met – histopathologic confirmation of the diagnosis is usually not needed.

Criteria 1, 2, and 4A are met – bronchoalveolar lavage or histopathologic confirmation of the diagnosis is not needed in a majority of these cases but may be important to allow decision making regarding management.

Criteria 1, 2A, 3, and 5 are met – these patients are usually identified as part of a case cluster. The index cases usually have more severe disease.

Criteria 2, 3, and 5 are met – in these cases, the diagnosis is first suspected after bronchoalveolar lavage or transbronchial lung biopsy.

Management

The mainstay of treatment is reduction of exposure to known irritants and secondarily about prevention and risk reduction.[93,95] If, after appropriate steps have been taken to remove the causative against from the environment or the patient from the environment and symptoms persist, then additional treatments may be indicated.

Treatment

Glucocorticoids are the medication of choice for severely affected patients based on clinical experience with patients suffering from farmer's lung and bird owner's lung. Prednisone, 0.5 mg to 1 mg per kilogram of ideal body weight daily, is the recommended dosage, maximum 60 mg daily.[96] There have been comparative studies of steroids with placebo and they have been shown to accelerate initial recovery, but no statistical significance was seen in the long-term outcomes. In severe refractory cases, lung transplants have been suggestive and 1 study found that there was a significant difference compared with those managed conservatively.[97]

Prognosis

Most patients with HP fully recover with conservative management and antigen avoidance. The rate of recovery depends on many different factors, such as specific antigen exposure, antigen load, and patient sensitivity. Bird owner's lung, for example, has been seen to take longer to recover and has an overall worse prognosis than farmer's lung. Patients who have had signs of pulmonary fibrosis have a worse prognosis than those who do not.[88]

REFERENCES

1. Gaffin J, Kanchongkittiphon W, Phipatanakul W. Perinatal and early childhood environmental factors influencing allergic asthma immunopathogenesis. Int Immunopharmacol 2014;22(1):21–30.
2. Kim H, Mazza J. Asthma. Allergy Asthma Clin Immunol 2011;7(Suppl 1):S2.
3. Abramson MJ, Puy RM, Weiner JM. Expert panel report 3 (EPR-3): guidelines for the diagnosis and management of asthma-summary report 2007. Injection allergen immunotherapy for asthma. Cochrane Database Syst Rev 2010;(8):CD001186.
4. Normansell R, Walker S, Milan SJ, et al. Omalizumab for asthma in adults and children. Cochrane Database Syst Rev 2014;(1):CD003559.
5. Romanet-Manent S, Charpin D, Magnan A, et al, EGEA Cooperative Group. Allergic vs nonallergic asthma: what makes the difference? Allergy 2002;57:607–13.
6. Gibeon D, Menzies-Gow A. Recent changes in the drug treatment of allergic asthma. Clin Med 2013;13(5):477–81.
7. Thomas M. Allergic rhinitis: evidence for impact on asthma [review]. BMC Pulm Med 2006;6(Suppl I):S4.
8. Mukherjee A, Zhang Z. Allergic asthma: influence of genetic and environmental factors. J Biol Chem 2011;286(38):32883–9.
9. Wark P, Murphy V, Mattes J. The interaction between mother and fetus and the development of allergic asthma. Expert Rev Respir Med 2014;8(1):57–66.
10. Hamelmann E, Gelfand E. IL-5 induced airway eosinophilia – the key to asthma? Immunol Rev 2001;179:182–91.
11. Boulay M, Boulet L. The relationships between atopy, rhinitis and asthma: pathophysiological considerations. Curr Opin Allergy Clin Immunol 2003;3:51–5.
12. Assayag M, Goldsein S, Samuni A, et al. Cyclic nitroxide radical attenuate inflammation and hyper-responsiveness in a mouse model of allergic asthma. Free Radic Biol Med 2015;87:148–56.
13. Afshar R, Medoff BD, Luster AD. Allergic asthma: a tale of many T cells. Clin Exp Allergy 2008;38:1847–57.
14. Hamelmann E, Tadeda K, Oshiba A, et al. Role of IgE in the development of allergic airway inflammation and airway hyperresponsiveness – a murine model. Allergy 1999;54:297–305.
15. Renauld J-C. New insights into the role of cytokines in asthma. J Clin Pathol 2001;54:577–89.
16. Frieri M. Advances in the understanding of allergic asthma. Allergy Asthma Proc 2007;28:614–9.
17. Kennedy JL, Heymann PW, Platts-Mills TAE. The role of allergy in severe asthma. Clin Exp Allergy 2012;42(5):659–69.
18. Brozek J, Bousquet J, Baena-Cagnani CE, et al. Allergic rhinitis and its impact on asthma (ARIA) guidelines. J Allergy Clin Immunol 2010;126(3):466–76.
19. Wright L. Environmental remediation in the treatment of allergy and asthma: latest updates. Curr Allergy Asthma Rep 2014;14(3):1–14.
20. Tilles S, Bardana E. Seasonal variation in bronchial hyperreactivity (BHR) in allergic patients. Clin Rev Allergy Immunol 1997;15:169–85.

21. Ma L, Zeng J, Mo B, et al. ANP/NPRA signaling preferentially mediates Th2 responses in favor of pathological processes during the course of acute allergic asthma. Int J Clin Exp Med 2015;8(4):5121–8.
22. Abramson MJ, Puy RM, Weiner JM. Injection allergen immunotherapy for asthma. Cochrane Database Syst Rev 2010;(8):CD001186.
23. Demoly P, Bousquet J, Michel F. Immunotherapy in allergic rhinitis: a prevention for asthma? Curr Probl Dermatol 1999;28:119–23.
24. Jaber R. Respiratory and allergic diseases: from upper respiratory tract infections to asthma. Prim Care 2002;29:231–61.
25. Greenberger PA. Allergic bronchopulmonary aspergillosis. J Allergy Clin Immunol 2002;110:685.
26. Tillie-Leblond I, Tonnel AB. Allergic bronchopulmonary aspergillosis. Allergy 2005;60:1004.
27. Agarwal R. Allergic bronchopulmonary aspergillosis. Chest 2009;135:805.
28. Patterson R, Greenberger PA, Radin RC, et al. Allergic bronchopulmonary aspergillosis: staging as an aid to management. Ann Intern Med 1982;96:286–91.
29. Hinson KF, Moon AJ, Plummer NS. Broncho-pulmonary aspergillosis: a review and a report of eight new cases. Thorax 1952;7:317–33.
30. Stevens DA, Moss RB, Kurup VP, et al. Allergic bronchopulmonary aspergillosis in cystic fibrosis–: state of the art. Cystic fibrosis foundation consensus conference. Clin Infect Dis 2003;37(Suppl 3):S225.
31. Riscili BP, Wood KL. Noninvasive pulmonary Aspergillus infections. Clin Chest Med 2009;30:315.
32. Greenberger PA, Smith LJ, Hsu CC, et al. Analysis of bronchoalveolar lavage in allergic bronchopulmonary aspergillosis: divergent responses of antigen-specific antibodies and total IgE. J Allergy Clin Immunol 1988;82:164.
33. Kauffman HF, Tomee JF, van der Werf TS, et al. Review of fungus- induced asthmatic reactions. Am J Respir Crit Care Med 1995;151:2109.
34. Chauhan B, Knutsen AP, Hutcheson PS, et al. T cell subsets, epitope mapping, and HLA-restriction in patients with allergic bronchopulmonary aspergillosis. J Clin Invest 1996;97:2324.
35. Kreindler JL, Steele C, Nguyen N, et al. Vitamin D3 attenuates Th2 responses to Aspergillus fumigatus mounted by CD4+ T cells from cystic fibrosis patients with allergic bronchopulmonary aspergillosis. J Clin Invest 2010;120:3242.
36. Gibson PG, Wark PA, Simpson JL, et al. Induced sputum IL-8 gene expression, neutrophil influx and MMP-9 in allergic bronchopulmonary aspergillosis. Eur Respir J 2003;21:582.
37. Agarwal R, Aggarwal AN, Gupta D, et al. Aspergillus hypersensitivity and allergic bronchopulmonary aspergillosis in patients with bronchial asthma: systematic review and meta- analysis. Int J Tuberc Lung Dis 2009;13:936.
38. Silverman M, Hobbs FD, Gordon IR, et al. Cystic fibrosis, atopy, and airways liability. Arch Dis Child 1978;53:873–7.
39. Schwartz HJ, Greenberger PA. The prevalence of allergic bronchopulmonary aspergillosis in patients with asthma, determined by serologic and radiologic criteria in patients at risk. J Lab Clin Med 1991;117:138–42.
40. Glancy JJ, Elder JL, McAleer R. Allergic bronchopulmonary fungal disease without clinical asthma. Thorax 1981;36:345–9.
41. Patterson R, Greenberger PA, Lee TM, et al. Prolonged evaluation of patients with corticosteroid-dependent asthma stage of allergic bronchopulmonary aspergillosis. J Allergy Clin Immunol 1987;80:663–8.

42. Radin RC, Greenberger PA, Patterson R, et al. Mold counts and exacerbations of allergic bronchopulmonary aspergillosis. Clin Allergy 1983;13:271–5.
43. Buckingham SJ, Hansell DM. Aspergillus in the lung: diverse and coincident forms. Eur Radiol 2003;13:1786.
44. Neeld DA, Goodman LR, Gurney JW, et al. Computerized tomography in the evaluation of allergic bronchopulmonary aspergillosis. Am Rev Respir Dis 1990;142: 1200–5.
45. Ward S, Heyneman L, Lee MJ, et al. Accuracy of CT in the diagnosis of allergic bronchopulmonary aspergillosis in asthmatic patients. AJR Am J Roentgenol 1999;173:937–42.
46. Mitchell TAM, Hamilos DL, Lynch DA, et al. Distribution and severity of bronchiectasis in allergic bronchopulmonary aspergillosis (ABPA). J Asthma 2000;37: 65–72.
47. Greenberger PA, Patterson R. Diagnosis and management of allergic bronchopulmonary aspergillosis. Ann Allergy 1986;56:444.
48. Paganin F, Trussard V, Seneterre E, et al. Chest radiography and high resolution computed tomography of the lungs in asthma. Am Rev Respir Dis 1992;146: 1084.
49. Angus RM, Davies ML, Cowan MD, et al. Computed tomographic scanning of the lung in patients with allergic bronchopulmonary aspergillosis and in asthmatic patients with a positive skin test to Aspergillus fumigatus. Thorax 1994;49:586.
50. Schuyler M, Cormier Y. The diagnosis of hypersensitivity pneumonitis. Chest 1997;111(3):534.
51. Kokkarinen JI, Tukiainen HO, Terho EO. Effect of corticosteroid treatment on the recovery of pulmonary function in farmer's lung. Am Rev Respir Dis 1992;145(1):3.
52. Lacasse Y, Selman M, Costabel U, et al, HP Study Group. Clinical diagnosis of hypersensitivity pneumonitis. Am J Respir Crit Care Med 2003;168(8):952.
53. Patel AM, Ryu JH, Reed CE. Hypersensitivity pneumonitis: current concepts and future questions. J Allergy Clin Immunol 2001;108(5):661.
54. Glazer CS, Rose CS, Lynch DA. Clinical and radiologic manifestations of hypersensitivity pneumonitis. J Thorac Imaging 2002;17(4):261.
55. Pérez-Padilla R, Salas J, Chapela R, et al. Mortality in Mexican patients with chronic pigeon breeder's lung compared with those with usual interstitial pneumonia. Am Rev Respir Dis 1993;148(1):49.
56. Walsh TJ, Anaissie EJ, Denning DW, et al. Treatment of aspergillosis: clinical practice guidelines of the Infectious Diseases Society of America. Clin Infect Dis 2008;46:327.
57. Ricketti AJ, Greenberger PA, Patterson R. Serum IgE as an important aid in management of allergic bronchopulmonary aspergillosis. J Allergy Clin Immunol 1984;74:68.
58. Wark PA, Hensley MJ, Saltos N, et al. Anti-inflammatory effect of itraconazole in stable allergic bronchopulmonary aspergillosis: a randomized controlled trial. J Allergy Clin Immunol 2003;111:952.
59. Lebrun-Vignes B, Archer VC, Diquet B, et al. Effect of itraconazole on the pharmacokinetics of prednisolone and methylprednisolone and cortisol secretion in healthy subjects. Br J Clin Pharmacol 2001;51:443.
60. Varis T, Kaukonen KM, Kivistö KT, et al. Plasma concentrations and effects of oral methylprednisolone are considerably increased by itraconazole. Clin Pharmacol Ther 1998;64:363.

61. Erwin GE, Fitzgerald JE. Case report: allergic bronchopulmonary aspergillosis and allergic fungal sinusitis successfully treated with voriconazole. J Asthma 2007;44:891.

62. Glackin L, Leen G, Elnazir B, et al. Voriconazole in the treatment of allergic bronchopulmonary aspergillosis in cystic fibrosis. Ir Med J 2009;102:29.

63. Chishimba L, Niven RM, Cooley J, et al. Voriconazole and posaconazole improve asthma severity in allergic bronchopulmonary aspergillosis and severe asthma with fungal sensitization. J Asthma 2012;49:423.

64. Knutsen AP, Bush RK, Demain JG, et al. Fungi and allergic lower respiratory tract diseases. J Allergy Clin Immunol 2012;129:280.

65. Rose C, King TE Jr. Controversies in hypersensitivity pneumonitis. Am Rev Respir Dis 1992;145(1):1.

66. Lopez M, Salvaggio JE. Epidemiology of hypersensitivity pneumonitis/allergic alveolitis. Monogr Allergy 1987;21:70.

67. Lalancette M, Carrier G, Laviolette M, et al. Farmer's lung. Long-term outcome and lack of predictive value of bronchoalveolar lavage fibrosing factors. Am Rev Respir Dis 1993;148(1):216.

68. Dalphin JC, Debieuvre D, Pernet D, et al. Prevalence and risk factors for chronic bronchitis and farmer's lung in French dairy farmers. Br J Ind Med 1993;50(10):941.

69. Grant IW, Blyth W, Wardrop VE, et al. Prevalence of farmer's lung in Scotland: a pilot survey. Br Med J 1972;1(5799):530.

70. Christensen LT, Schmidt CD, Robbins L. Pigeon breeders' disease–a prevalence study and review. Clin Allergy 1975;5(4):417.

71. Murin S, Bilello KS, Matthay R. Other smoking-affected pulmonary diseases. Clin Chest Med 2000;21(1):121.

72. Solaymani-Dodaran M, West J, Smith C, et al. Extrinsic allergic alveolitis: incidence and mortality in the general population. QJM 2007;100(4):233.

73. McSharry C, Banham SW, Boyd G. Effect of cigarette smoking on the antibody response to inhaled antigens and the prevalence of extrinsic allergic alveolitis among pigeon breeders. Clin Allergy 1985;15(5):487.

74. Salvaggio JE. The identification of hypersensitivity pneumonitis. Hosp Pract (1995) 1995;30(5):57.

75. Reynolds HY. Hypersensitivity pneumonitis. Clin Chest Med 1982;3(3):503.

76. Alegre J, Morell F, Cobo E. Respiratory symptoms and pulmonary function of workers exposed to cork dust, toluene diisocyanate and conidia. Scand J Work Environ Health 1990;16(3):175.

77. Zamarrón C, del Campo F, Paredes C. Extrinsic allergic alveolitis due to exposure to esparto dust. J Intern Med 1992;232(2):177.

78. Bernstein DI, Lummus ZL, Santilli G, et al. Machine operator's lung. A hypersensitivity pneumonitis disorder associated with exposure to metalworking fluid aerosols. Chest 1995;108(3):636.

79. Ganier M, Lieberman P, Fink J, et al. Humidifier lung. An outbreak in office workers. Chest 1980;77(2):183.

80. Rose CS, Martyny JW, Newman LS, et al. "Lifeguard lung": endemic granulomatous pneumonitis in an indoor swimming pool. Am J Public Health 1998;88(12):1795.

81. Simpson C, Garabrant D, Torrey S, et al. Hypersensitivity pneumonitis-like reaction and occupational asthma associated with 1,3-bis(isocyanatomethyl) cyclohexane pre-polymer. Am J Ind Med 1996;30(1):48.

82. Banaszak EF, Thiede WH, Fink JN. Hypersensitivity pneumonitis due to contamination of an air conditioner. N Engl J Med 1970;283(6):271.
83. Schwarz MI, King TE Jr, editors. Interstitial lung disease. 5th edition. Shelton (CT): People's Medical Publishing House; 2011.
84. Agostini C, Trentin L, Facco M, et al. New aspects of hypersensitivity pneumonitis. Curr Opin Pulm Med 2004;10(5):378.
85. Schlueter DP. Response of the lung to inhaled antigens. Am J Med 1974;57(3):476.
86. Allen DH, Williams GV, Woolcock AJ. Bird breeder's hypersensitivity pneumonitis: progress studies of lung function after cessation of exposure to the provoking antigen. Am Rev Respir Dis 1976;114(3):555.
87. Zacharisen MC, Schlueter DP, Kurup VP, et al. The long-term outcome in acute, subacute, and chronic forms of pigeon breeder's disease hypersensitivity pneumonitis. Ann Allergy Asthma Immunol 2002;88(2):175.
88. Vourlekis JS, Schwarz MI, Cherniack RM, et al. The effect of pulmonary fibrosis on survival in patients with hypersensitivity pneumonitis. Am J Med 2004; 116(10):662.
89. Buschman DL, Gamsu G, Waldron JA Jr, et al. Chronic hypersensitivity pneumonitis: use of CT in diagnosis. AJR Am J Roentgenol 1992;159(5):957.
90. Cormier Y, Lacasse Y. Keys to the diagnosis of hypersensitivity pneumonitis: the role of serum precipitins, lung biopsy, and high-resolution computed tomography. Clin Pulm Med 1996;3:72.
91. Richerson HB, Bernstein IL, Fink JN, et al. Guidelines for the clinical evaluation of hypersensitivity pneumonitis. Report of the subcommittee on hypersensitivity pneumonitis. J Allergy Clin Immunol 1989;84(5 Pt 2):839.
92. Terho EO. Diagnostic criteria for farmer's lung. Am J Ind Med 1986;10:329.
93. Rose CS. Water-related lung diseases. Occup Med 1992;7(2):271.
94. Muilenberg ML. Aeroallergen assessment by microscopy and culture. Immunol Allergy Clin N Am 1989;9:245.
95. Cormier Y, Bélanger J. Long-term physiologic outcome after acute farmer's lung. Chest 1985;87(6):796.
96. Mönkäre S. Influence of corticosteroid treatment on the course of farmer's lung. Eur J Respir Dis 1983;64(4):283.
97. Kern RM, Singer JP, Koth L, et al. Lung transplantation for hypersensitivity pneumonitis. Chest 2015;147(6):1558–65.

Insect Allergy

Hobart Lee, MD*, Sara Halverson, MD, Regina Mackey, MD

KEYWORDS

- Insect bites • Insect stings • Diagnosis • Treatment • Allergic reaction
- Anaphylaxis • Venom immunotherapy

KEY POINTS

- Insect bites and stings are common and mostly clinically mild, but providers should be aware of potential systemic reactions, including anaphylaxis.
- Common insects that bite or sting include mosquitoes, ticks, flies, fleas, biting midges, bees, and wasps; immunocompromised patients or patients with hypersensitivity reactions may experience large local reactions or papular urticaria.
- The key to diagnosis is a thorough clinical history and identification of the insect when possible; skin testing and serum immunoglobulin E levels are indicated for certain high risk patients.
- Management of insect bites or stings is usually supportive care with antihistamines, pain medications, and cold compresses; patient with anaphylaxis should be given epinephrine and transported to the emergency department.
- Venom immunotherapy (VIT) can be helpful for patients with anaphylaxis or risk for severe reactions; VIT is highly effective in reducing the risk of future reactions.

INTRODUCTION

The purpose of this article is to review the current available material pertaining to insect bites and stings. It will review the development, presentation, and treatment of both common insect bites and insect stings. Although the clinical presentation may be similar between insect bites and insect stings, the evaluation and treatment can differ considerably. The proper diagnosis and treatment can decrease the risk of complications, which can include life-threatening anaphylaxis.

BACKGROUND

Insects are arthropod invertebrates characterized by an exoskeleton and a 3-part body with 3 pairs of jointed legs. There are an estimated 4 to 6 million species of insects,[1] which represent over 50% of all living organisms on earth.[2] Insect bites and

Department of Family Medicine, Loma Linda University, 25455 Barton Road, Suite 209B, Loma Linda, CA 92354, USA
* Corresponding author.
E-mail address: holee@llu.edu

Prim Care Clin Office Pract 43 (2016) 417–431
http://dx.doi.org/10.1016/j.pop.2016.04.010
primarycare.theclinics.com
0095-4543/16/$ – see front matter © 2016 Elsevier Inc. All rights reserved.

stings are common and generally clinically mild, but can lead to serious medical conditions, including life-threatening complications. Common insects that bite include: bedbugs, chiggers, fleas, flies, mosquitoes, and ticks. Common insect stings, involving in the introduction of venom into people, include ants, bees, and centipedes.

EPIDEMIOLOGY

Exact incidence statistics on insect bites or stings is unknown, as most people bitten or stung have mild local reactions that are not reported or tracked. In Europe, between 56% and 94% of people report being stung by a Hymenoptera insect.[3] The prevalence of systemic reactions to Hymenoptera stings is reported to be 0.5% to 3.3% in adults and 0.15% to .8% in children.[4] In Florida, review of emergency department billing codes suggests that 42% of pediatric patients experienced systemic reactions to Hymenoptera stings.[5]

Among stinging ant endemic areas of the United States, 55% of people reported being stung within a 3-week period.[3] The prevalence, however, of systemic anaphylaxis to ant stings is reported to be less than 1%.[6]

Approximately 40 to 100 Americans die annually from insect bites or stings, although many experts believe the true mortality is higher.[7]

RISK FACTORS

Risk factors for insect bites and stings are related strongly to environmental exposure. People who live next to bodies of water or wetlands are at risk for mosquitoes, biting midges, or other insects that require nearby water to reproduce. Living near wooded or grassy areas is a risk factor for tick bites. People who work with or live with animals, particularly horses, dogs, or cats are at risk for fly or flea bites. Finally, occupational hazards like gardening or beekeeping increase the risk for insect-specific bites or stings. Seasonal exacerbation of papular urticaria may occur, related to the reexposure of the insect.[8]

CLINICAL PRESENTATION

Insect bites and stings typically result in mild, local, allergic reactions. Delayed hypersensitivity and systemic reactions including anaphylaxis are rare but may occur. Most insect bites and stings result in a local inflammatory response at the specific site. Large areas of redness, itching, and swelling mimicking cellulitis may occur.[9] Vesicular or bullous lesions may also arise (**Fig. 1**).[10]

One common response to insect bite or stings is papular urticaria (**Table 1**). This insect bite-induced hypersensitivity reaction is common in children ages 2 to 10, but can occur in adolescents and adults. Common insect culprits include mites, ticks, fleas, mosquitoes, and flies. Typically, papular urticaria presents as recurrent erythematous, pruritic papules from 3 to 10 mm in size, with possible vesicles and wheals. Papular urticaria often occurs in a line or grouped in clusters. Extremities and clothing-constricted areas like ankles and waistbands are common presenting areas for papular urticaria. Genital, perianal, and axillary regions are not usually involved.[8,11]

Immunocompromised patients, including those with human immunodeficiency virus (HIV) or cancer, may develop more severe local allergic reactions and systemic signs, including fever, malaise, headache, and lymphadenopathy (**Fig. 2**).[12,13] Some patients may develop these systematic symptoms and signs without being immunocompromised. In severe cases, insect bites and stings may cause anaphylaxis, "a severe, potentially fatal, systemic allergic reaction that occurs suddenly after contact with

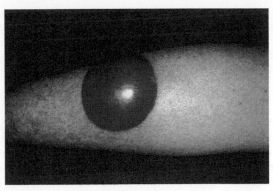

Fig. 1. A large bullous reaction to a fire ant bite on the arm. (*Courtesy of* Mark Lebwohl, MD, Mount Sinai Hospital, New York, NY.)

Table 1
Distribution of papular urticaria as a diagnostic tool

Arthropod	Exposed Area	Ventral Surfaces	Constricting Band (Waist, Sock)	Generalized
Mosquito	Yes	No	No	No
Flies	Yes	No	No	No
Gnats	Yes	No	No	No
Scabies	Yes	No	No	No
Other mites	Yes	Yes	Yes	No
Ticks	No	No	Yes	No
Lepidoptera	Yes	No	Yes	No

(*From* Demain JG. Papular urticaria and things that bite in the night. Curr Allergy Asthma Rep 2003;3(4):291–303; with permission.)

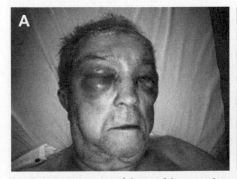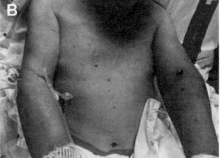

Fig. 2. An exaggerated insect bite reaction on the eye, forehead (*A*), and arm (*B*) of a chronic lymphatic leukemia patient. (*From* Royo-Cebrecos C, Garcia-Vidal C. Exaggerated insect bite reaction related to chronic leukemia. Mayo Clin Proc 2013;88(4):e37; with permission.)

an allergy-causing substance."[14] Criteria for diagnosing anaphylaxis can be found in **Box 1**. The key clinical symptoms include rapid onset, involvement of skin or mucosa, along with cardiovascular or respiratory symptoms. Patients with mast cell disease must be carefully assessed for analphylaxis after insect bites and stings, especially after bee or wasp stings.[15]

MOSQUITOES

Mosquitoes belong to the order Diptera and family Culicidae. They are among the most common insect bites. Symptoms include local swelling, warmth, erthyema, pain, and pruritis with accompanying papules and wheals. Some patients may experience larger local reactions with ecchymosis or vesicular lesions accompanied by systemic symptoms including fever, generalized urticaria, wheezing, and angioedema (**Fig. 3**). A serum sickness-like condition and anaphylaxis have also been reported.[9,16,17]

TICKS

Tick bites without secondary infection typically cause a local allergic reaction characterized by erythematous, papular lesions accompanied by pain and pruritis, which can persist up to weeks after the initial bite. Hard ticks are found in brush fields and tall

---

Box 1
Clinical criteria for diagnosing anaphylaxis

Anaphylaxis is highly likely when any of the following 3 criteria are fulfilled:

1. Acute onset of an illness (minutes to several hours) with involvement of the skin, mucosal tissue, or both (eg, generalized hives, pruritus or flushing, swollen lips-tongue-uvula) and at least 1 of the following
   a. Respiratory compromise (eg, dyspnea, wheeze–bronchospasm, stridor, reduced peak expiratory flow (PEF), hypoxemia)
   b. Reduced blood pressure or associated symptoms of end–organ dysfunction (eg, hypotonia [collapse], syncope, incontinence)

2. At least 2 of the following that occur rapidly after exposure to a likely allergen for that patient (minutes to several hours):
   a. Involvement of the skin–mucosal tissue (eg, generalized hives, itch–flush, swollen lips-tongue-uvula)
   b. Respiratory compromise (eg, dyspnea, wheeze–bronchospasm, stridor, reduced PEF, hypoxemia)
   c. Reduced BP or associated symptoms (eg, hypotonia [collapse], syncope, incontinence)
   d. Persistent gastrointestinal symptoms (eg, crampy abdominal pain, vomiting)

3. Reduced blood pressure after exposure to known allergen for that patient (minutes to several hours):
   a. Infants and children: low systolic blood pressure (age specific) or greater than 30% decrease in systolic blood pressure[a]
   b. Adults: systolic blood pressure of less than 90 mm Hg or greater than 30% decrease from that person's baseline

[a] Low systolic blood pressure for children is defined as less than 70 mm Hg from 1 month to 1 year, less than 70 mm Hg + (2 × age) from 1 to 10 years, and less than 90 mm Hg from 11 to 17 years.
From Sampson HA, Munoz-Fulong A, Campbell RL, et al. Second symposium on the definition and management of anaphylaxis: summary report: Second National Institute of Allergy and Infectious Disease/Food Allergy and Anaphylaxis Network Symposium. J Allergy Clin Immunol 2006;117:393; with permission.

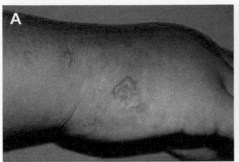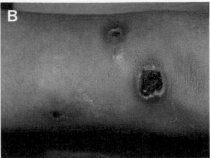

Fig. 3. Typical skin lesions in a patient with hypersensitivity to mosquito bites. (*A*) erythema and swelling with blister formation 2 days after the mosquito bites. (*B*) skin necrosis and ulcer formation after 10 days. (*From* Asada H. Hypersensitivity to mosquito bites: a unique pathogenic mechanism linking Epstein-Barr virus infection, allergy and oncogenesis. J Dermatol Sci 2007;45(3):154; with permission.)

grass and then attach to people and can feed for days (**Fig. 4**).[18] Eight percent to 16% of patients can experience anaphylactic symptoms depending on the type of tick and previous tick exposure.[19–21]

FLIES

Several fly species are able to bite people and cause local inflammatory reactions (**Fig. 5**). These include black flies, deer flies, horse flies, and sand flies. Most patients will complain of painful bites with local inflammatory reactions similar to other insect bites described previously. Case reports of anaphylaxis have been reported with horse fly bites.[22,23]

FLEAS

Flea bites create erythematous papules and can also lead to papular urticaria,[24] because the bites are pruritic and excoriation of the papules or vesicles are common. Large bullae have been reported as well.[25] Fleas usually transfer from animals such as dog or cats.[18]

BITING MIDGES

Biting midges are tiny biting flies. Due to their small size and painful bite, they go by other colloquial names, including, punkies, no-see-ums, flying teeth, and no-nos. Midges prefer low light, and females feed at sunrise and sunset. Water is necessary for their life cycle, so oceans and wetlands are common areas to find biting midges. Their bites can create papules, wheals from 2 to 10 cm in size, or honey-crusted lesions due to excoriations, which can persist from weeks to months.[26,27]

BEE AND WASP STINGS

Bees belong to the order Hymenoptera, including bees, yellow jackets, hornets, wasps, and stinging ants (**Figs. 6** and **7**). The most common local reactions include pain, erythema, swelling and pruritis. Large swelling over 10 cm is possible, and is associated with an increased risk for systemic reactions upon repeat exposure. Moderate systematic symptoms include mild asthma, moderate angioedema, and

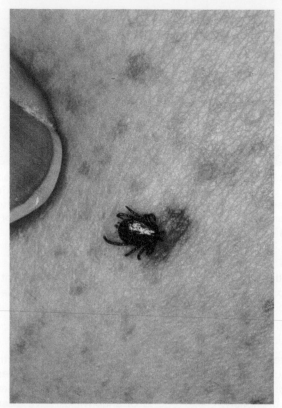

Fig. 4. Dermacentor tick feeding on skin. (*From* Steen CJ, Carbonaro PA, Schwartz RA. Arthropods in dermatology. J Am Acad Dermatol 2004;50(6):828; with permission.)

abdominal pain with vomiting, diarrhea, and dizziness. More severe systemic symptoms include respiratory difficulty, hypotension, loss of consciousness, or seizures.[28]

DIAGNOSIS

The accurate diagnosis of insect allergy requires a careful and detailed history, including prior exposure to bites and stings and potential venom allergy. The 1

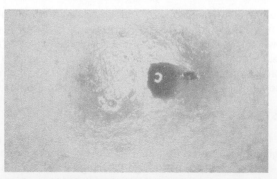

Fig. 5. Wound myiasis from a botfly. (*From* Demain JG. Papular urticaria and things that bite in the night. Curr Allergy Asthma Rep 2003;3(4):298; with permission.)

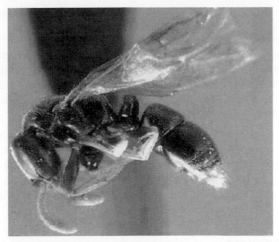

Fig. 6. Female winged reproductive Hypoponera genus. Females are approximately 2.7 to 2.9 mm in length. (*From* Klotz JH, deShazo RD, Pinnas JL, et al. Adverse reactions to ants other than imported fire ants. Ann Allergy Asthma Immunol 2005;95(5):422; with permission.)

exception to a clinical diagnosis is the specific diagnosis of Hymenoptera allergy, which is based upon the clinical history and the presence of venom-specific immunoglobulin E (IgE) antibodies.[29-32]

MEDICAL HISTORY

A detailed medical history is the most important and key to a proper diagnosis. Usually the sting or bite is painful, and patients are aware of the onset.[31]

Questions to consider include:

- When did the bite or sting episode happen?
- How many bites or stings did you get?
- Where did you get bitten or stung?

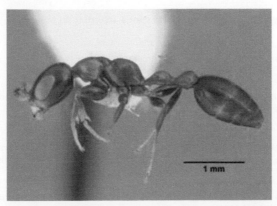

1 mm

Fig. 7. Worker ant from Psuedomyrmex ejectus. (*From* Klotz JH, deShazo RD, Pinnas JL, et al. Adverse reactions to ants other than imported fire ants. Ann Allergy Asthma Immunol 2005;95(5):423; with permission.)

- After the bite or sting, how long before other symptoms appeared? Did you have any symptoms that appeared later on?
- How did you treat the bite or sting?
- Have you ever been bitten or stung before? What was the reaction to those prior episodes? (a large location reaction is an area of redness or swelling that enlarges of 2 days, is usually >10 cm in size, and resolves in 5–10 days)
- Do you have a regular exposure to insects from either your occupation or recreational activities?

A thorough review of symptoms should be done, including assessing for shortness of breath, palpitations, dizziness, or lightheadedness. Medications that can exaggerate the immune response, such as angiotensin-converting enzyme (ACE) inhibitors, or beta-blockers, should be assessed. If the patient accessed emergency services, medical records should be obtained for review. Patients with systemic reactions should be graded by severity (**Boxes 2** and **3**).

IDENTIFICATION OF INSECT

The history can provide important clues to identifying the possible insect. For example, yellow jackets tend to be found near garbage or food. The season of year can also be helpful: honey bee stings tend to occur in the spring and summer, while vespid stings occur more frequently in late summer and fall. If the patient cannot describe the insect in question, it can sometimes be identified based on the patient's geographic location or setting where the bite or sting occurred.

Patients should be encouraged to bring in the insect, when available, for physician identification.[28] Physicians can use a reference book or internet resources (http://www.cdc.gov/niosh/topics/insects/) to help identify the insect.

Some key distinguishing factors include[33] bumble bees, honey bees, hornets, and wasps.

Bumble bees (Bombus spp) have abundant feathering and yellow, orange, or white stripes on the thorax and abdomen. They are slow, fly low to the ground, and make a characteristic loud buzzing sound. Ordinarily, bumble bees are calm insects and only sting in extreme situations like when their nest is attacked.

Box 2
Classification of systemic reactions to insect stings according to Mueller

Grade I

Generalized urticaria, itching, malaise, and anxiety

Grade II

Any of the previously mentioned symptoms plus at least 2 of the following: angioedema, chest constriction, nausea, vomiting, diarrhea, abdominal pain, dizziness

Grade III

Any of the previously mentioned symptoms plus at least 2 of the following: dyspnea, wheezing, stridor, dysarthria, hoarseness, weakness, confusion, feeling of impending disaster

Grade IV

Any of the previously described symptoms plus at least 2 of the following: fall in blood pressure, collapse, loss of consciousness, incontinence, cyanosis

From Mueller HL. Diagnosis and treatment of insect sensitivity. J Asthma Res 1966;3(4):331–3.

Box 3
Classification of systemic reactions modified according to Ring and Messmer
Grade I
Generalized skin symptoms (eg, flush, generalized urticaria, angioedema)
Grade II
Mild-to-moderate pulmonary, cardiovascular, and/or gastrointestinal symptoms
Grade III
Anaphylactic shock, loss of consciousness
Grade IV
Cardiac arrest, apnea
From Ring J, Messmer K. Incidence and severity of anaphylactoid reactions to colloid volume substitutes. Lancet 1977;1(8009):466–9.

Honey bees (Apis mellifera) are nearly uniform dark brown color. After a bee sting, the bee leaves the entire stinging apparatus with venom reservoir in the skin (**Fig. 8**). This kind of sting often happen near beehives or orchards (**Fig. 9**).

Hornets (Vespa) build their nests in hollow attics and trees. In contrast to honey bees, they do not leave their stinger in the skin.

Wasps (Vespidae) have a black-yellow or dark brown-yellow color. Some wasps build their nests in the ground, and others build them in tree branches or attics. Like hornets, they do not leave the venom apparatus in the skin. Wasps are attracted to sweet food and drinks in open-air environments (see **Fig. 9**).

DIAGNOSTIC TESTS

The 2011 stinging insect hypersensitivity practice parameters provide guidance on when to perform diagnostic tests.[28] Patients who experience a systemic allergic reaction after an insect bite or sting are at increased risk for subsequent systemic reaction,

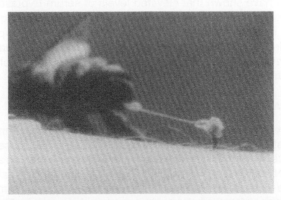

Fig. 8. Honeybee sting embedded in human skin. (*From* Schumacher MJ, Tveten MS, Egen NB. Rate and quantity of delivery of venom from honeybee stings. J Allergy Clin Immunol 1994;93(5):832; with permission.)

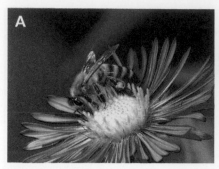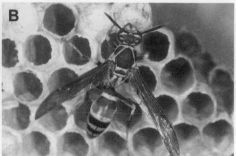

Fig. 9. (*A*) the honeybee *(Apis mellifera);* and (*B*) a common species of wasp (*Polistes exclamans*). (*From* Golden DB. Insect sting allergy and venom immunotherapy: a model and a mystery. J Allergy Clin Immunol 2005;115(3):441; with permission.)

and diagnostic testing should be performed.[33] A referral to an allergist–immunologist is recommended when a person:

- Experiences a systemic allergic reaction to an insect sting
- Develops a systemic allergic reaction in which an insect sting could be the cause
- Needs education regarding stinging avoidance or treatment in case of emergency
- Might be candidate for venom immunotherapy (VIT)
- Has a coexisting situation that may complicate the treatment of the allergic reaction (eg, epinephrine in patients with cardiac disease)

Diagnosis usually starts with hypersensitivity skin testing, indicated for people who are candidates for VIT.

Skin testing should be used for initial measurement of the venom-specific IgE. If the skin test response is negative and the patient has had a severe allergic reaction, further testing, such as repeat skin testing or in vivo testing, can be done.

In patients with severe skin disease or dermatographism or in patients who cannot undergo skin testing, in vitro testing using enzyme-linked immunosorbent assay (ELISA) or radioallergosorbent test (RAST) techniques can detect venom-specific IgE antibodies. The sensitivity of in vitro tests was 88.5% for wasps and 94% for bee venom.[33]

Recent studies have shown that elevated levels of serum tryptase are associated with a high risk of severe anaphylaxis following a subsequent sting. Tryptase is an enzyme present in mast cell granules and basophils. Elevated tryptase levels can be useful in confirming a diagnosis of anaphylaxis that is not food related. It is recommended to determine serum tryptase in patients with a severe anaphylactic reaction after a bite or sting.[28,33]

DIFFERENTIAL DIAGNOSIS

Although not covered in this article, several important diseases are transmitted through insect bites and stings. Mosquitos serve as vectors for several diseases, including chikungunya, dengue hemorrhagic fever, malaria, LaCrosse encephalitis and St. Louis encephalitis, West Nile virus, and yellow fever. Tick bites can transmit babesiosis, human ehrlichosis, Lyme disease, Rocky Mountain spotted fever, and tularemia. Fly bites can lead to bartonellosis, leishmaniasis, myiasis, and onchocerciasis. Fleas can transmit bartonellosis, the plague, tungiasis, and typhus. Biting midges can lead to filarial worm infections. It is important to assess for these secondary infections when indicated.

An allergic reaction and anaphylaxis can be triggered in numerous ways, but the 3 most common triggers are insect bites or stings, food, and medication. Some other entities causing skin allergic reaction with or without systemic involvement can resemble insect allergic reaction. Other common diagnoses that can mimic an insect bite or sting include angioedema, cellulitis, cat scratch disease, and animal bites.

MANAGEMENT/TREATMENT

An overview algorithm for management of an insect bite or sting is found in **Fig. 10**. For local insect bite or sting reactions (eg, redness, swelling, itching, and pain), symptomatic treatment with oral antihistamines, pain medications, and cold compresses is recommended. Early removal of the stinger might decrease additional injection of venom. Ninety percent of venom delivery is complete within 20 seconds, so intervention is only helpful if it occurs immediately.[28,34]

Large local reactions increase in size over 24 to 48 hours, cause swelling beyond the immediate sting area, and can take 5 to 10 days to resolve. Up to 10% of patients with large local reactions may have future systemic reactions, and providers should consider prescribing injectable epinephrine as a precaution. Oral corticosteroids are also sometimes used to decrease swelling. Antibiotics are not helpful for these allergic reactions. VIT is not recommended for large local reactions unless these reactions become a frequent occurrence and the patient has detectable immediate hypersensitivity skin test or in vitro tests for serum-specific IgE.[28]

Systemic reactions can include almost any body system. When anaphylaxis is present, the patient should be treated immediately with injectable epinephrine and transported to the emergency department. Once in the emergency department, a patient not responding to epinephrine injection should be given an intravenous infusion of epinephrine. Patients should be kept supine, and adjunctive antihistamines and corticosteroids can also be given, but never as substitute for epinephrine. Airway and blood pressure support should be given; patients should be observed for at least 4 to 8 hours, longer if any history of risk factors for severe anaphylaxis such as asthma, biphasic reactions, or protracted anaphylaxis exists. Elevated tryptase levels have also been associated with systemic reactions to VIT and greater failure rates with more frequent relapse after immunotherapy has been stopped. After discharge from the emergency department, patients with anaphylaxis should be seen by an allergist–immunologist.[28,35–37]

A rare allergic reaction is serum sickness, which involves fever, malaise, urticarial, and arthralgia starting several days after an insect sting. This can increase risk of future anaphylaxis, so VIT is appropriate in these patients.[38,39]

Besides venom injection from stinging insects, other insect-related allergic reactions, exist including a severe reaction to mosquito bites called skeeter syndrome, a large local reaction or systemic reaction with low-grade fever that can require both supportive treatment and possibly oral glucocorticoids and epinephrine and transport to the emergency department when anaphylaxis is present.[9,34]

A more unusual source of insect allergy has been reported in cases of hymenoptera venom exposure via ingestion of wine or grape juice causing systemic symptoms.[40]

PREVENTION: VENOM IMMUNOTHERAPY

For patients who have had systemic reactions to a stinging insect or fire ant, VIT may be an option to help decrease the risk of future severe reactions. The criteria for immunotherapy include evidence of specific IgE antibodies to the offending insect in a patient who has had a systemic reaction. Patients under the age of 16 with only

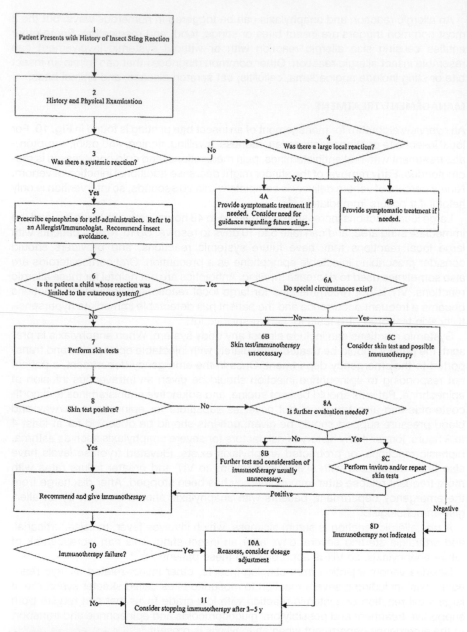

Fig. 10. Algorithm for management of stinging insect reactions. (*From* Golden DB, Moffitt J, Nicklas RA, et al. Stinging insect hypersensitivity: a practice parameter update 2011. J Allergy Clin Immunol 2011;127(4):854.e20; with permission.)

cutaneous symptoms do not need immunotherapy.[35] High-risk pregnant patients may be considered for VIT.[4]

Protocols vary depending on inciting insect (honeybee vs vespid vs fire ant) and how quickly to reach maintenance dosing. Initial doses are given 1 to 2 times per week, and the standard (slow) protocol recommends reaching maintenance dosing in 8 to 15 weeks.

Ultrarush protocols with possible hospitalization (1–2 days) may be used but also increase the risk of an adverse reaction.[4,28] VIT is highly effective in reducing the risk of large local reactions or systematic reactions with a number needed to treat 2-4 patients.[41] ACE inhibitor use, honeybee VIT, adverse reactions during VIT, and increased tryptase levels are all associated with risk of VIT failure.[42] Large local reactions, serum sickness, and anaphylaxis are all reported adverse effects from VIT.[4,28] Premedication with antihistamines may reduce local and mild systemic adverse reactions. Patients should be kept in the office at least 30 minutes to be observed after an immunotherapy injection. The risk of systemic reaction per injection is about 0.2%.[43] Life-threatening anaphylaxis is rarely seen after 30 minutes. VIT is recommended for 3 to 5 years or sooner if skin testing becomes negative or IgE levels return to normal. Some experts recommend indefinite treatment for certain patients.[28]

REFERENCES

1. Novotny V, Basset Y, Miller SE, et al. Low host specificity of herbivorous insects in a tropical forest. Nature 2002;416(6883):841–4.

2. Threats to global diversity. Available at: http://www.globalchange.umich.edu/globalchange2/current/lectures/biodiversity/biodiversity.html. Accessed October 11, 2015.

3. Antonicelli L, Bilò MB, Bonifazi F. Epidemiology of hymenoptera allergy. Curr Opin Allergy Clin Immunol 2002;2(4):341–6.

4. Pesek RD, Lockey RF. Treatment of Hymenoptera venom allergy: an update. Curr Opin Allergy Clin Immunol 2014;14(4):340–6.

5. Bilò BM, Bonifazi F. Epidemiology of insect-venom anaphylaxis. Curr Opin Allergy Clin Immunol 2008;8(4):330–7.

6. deShazo RD, Butcher BT, Banks WA. Reactions to the stings of the imported fire ant. N Engl J Med 1990;323:462–6.

7. Clark S, Camargo CA Jr. Emergency treatment and prevention of insect-sting anaphylaxis. Curr Opin Allergy Clin Immunol 2006;6(4):279–83.

8. Demain JG. Papular urticaria and things that bite in the night. Curr Allergy Asthma Rep 2003;3(4):291–303.

9. Simons FE, Peng Z. Skeeter syndrome. J Allergy Clin Immunol 1999;104(3):705–7.

10. Vassallo C, Passamonti F, Cananzi R, et al. Exaggerated insect bite-like reaction in patients affected by oncohaematological diseases. Acta Derm Venereol 2005;85(1):76–7.

11. Hernandez RG, Cohen BA. Insect bite-induced hypersensitivity and the SCRATCH principles: a new approach to papular urticaria. Pediatrics 2006;118(1):e189–96.

12. Royo-Cebrecos C, Garcia-Vidal C. Exaggerated insect bite reaction related to chronic leukemia. Mayo Clin Proc 2013;88(4):e37.

13. Smith KJ, Skelton HG 3rd, Vogel P, et al. Exaggerated insect bite reactions in patients positive for HIV. Military Medical Consortium for the Advancement of Retroviral Research. J Am Acad Dermatol 1993;29(2):269–72.

14. Sampson HA, Munoz-Fulong A, Campbell RL, et al. Second symposium on the definition and management of anaphylaxis: summary report: Second National Institute of Allergy and Infectious Disease/Food Allergy and Anaphylaxis Network Symposium. J Allergy Clin Immunol 2006;117:391–7.

15. Bonadonna P, Perbellini O, Passalacqua G, et al. Clonal mast cell disorders in patients with systemic reactions to Hymenoptera stings and increased serum tryptase levels. J Allergy Clin Immunol 2009;123(3):680–6.
16. Przybilla B, Ruëff F. Insect stings: clinical features and management. Dtsch Arztebl Int 2012;109(13):238–48.
17. Peng Z, Ho MK, Li C, et al. Evidence for natural desensitization to mosquito salivary allergens: mosquito saliva specific IgE and IgG levels in children. Ann Allergy Asthma Immunol 2004;93(6):553–6.
18. Juckett G. Arthropod Bites. Am Fam Physician 2013;88(12):841–7.
19. Kleine-Tebbe J, Heinatz A, Gräser I, et al. Bites of the European pigeon tick (Argas reflexus): risk of IgE-mediated sensitizations and anaphylactic reactions. J Allergy Clin Immunol 2006;117(1):190–5.
20. Gauci M, Loh RK, Stone BF, et al. Allergic reactions to the Australian paralysis tick, Ixodes holocyclus: diagnostic evaluation by skin test and radioimmunoassay. Clin Exp Allergy 1989;19(3):279–83.
21. Moneret-Vautrin DA, Beaudouin E, Kanny G, et al. Anaphylactic shock caused by ticks (Ixodes ricinus). J Allergy Clin Immunol 1998;101(1):144–5.
22. Hemmer W, Focke M, Vieluf D, et al. Anaphylaxis induced by horsefly bites: identification of a 69 kd IgE-binding salivary gland protein from Chrysops spp. (Diptera, Tabanidae) by western blot analysis. J Allergy Clin Immunol 1998; 101(1):134–6.
23. Freye HB, Litwin C. Coexistent anaphylaxis to diptera and hymenoptera. Ann Allergy Asthma Immunol 1996;76(3):270–2.
24. Naimer SA, Cohen AD, Mumcuoglu KY, et al. Household papular urticaria. Isr Med Assoc J 2002;4(11):911–3.
25. Golomb MR, Golomb HS. What's eating you? Cat flea (Ctenocephalides felis). Cutis 2010;85(1):10–1.
26. Cohn BA. Biting midges–those marauding "no-see-ums". Int J Dermatol 2003; 42(6):459–60.
27. Chen YH, Lee MF, Lan JL, et al. Hypersensitivity to Forcipomyia taiwana (biting midge): clinical analysis and identification of major For t 1, For t 2 and For t 3 allergens. Allergy 2005;60:1518–23.
28. Golden DB, Moffitt J, Nicklas RA, et al. Joint Task Force on Practice Parameters, American Academy of Allergy, Asthma & Immunology (AAAAI), American College of Allergy, Asthma & Immunology (ACAAI), Joint Council of Allergy, Asthma and Immunology. Stinging insect hypersensitivity: a practice parameter update 2011. J Allergy Clin Immunol 2011;127(4):852–4.e1–23.
29. Demain JG, Minaei AA, Tracy JM. Anaphylaxis and insect allergy. Curr Opin Allergy Clin Immunol 2010;10(4):318–22.
30. Scherer K, Bircher AJ, Heijnen IA. Diagnosis of stinging insect allergy: utility of cellular in-vitro tests. Curr Opin Allergy Clin Immunol 2009;9(4):343–50.
31. Biló BM, Rueff F, Mosbech H, et al. Diagnosis of Hymenoptera venom allergy. Allergy 2005;60(11):1339–49.
32. Tracy JM, Khan FS, Demain JG. Insect anaphylaxis: where are we? The stinging facts 2012. Curr Opin Allergy Clin Immunol 2012;12(4):400–5.
33. Matysiak J, Matysiak J, Bręborowicz A, et al. Diagnosis of hymenoptera venom allergy–with special emphasis on honeybee (Apis mellifera) venom allergy. Ann Agric Environ Med 2013;20(4):875–9.
34. Schumacher MJ, Tveten MS, Egen NB. Rate and quantity of delivery of venom from honeybee stings. J Allergy Clin Immunol 1994;93(5):831–5.

35. Cox L, Nelson H, Lockey R, et al. Allergen immunotherapy: a practice parameter third update. J Allergy Clin Immunol 2011;127(1 Suppl):S1–55.
36. Lieberman P, Nicklas RA, Oppenheimer J, et al. The diagnosis and management of anaphylaxis practice parameter: 2010 update. J Allergy Clin Immunol 2010; 126(3):477–80.e1–42.
37. Campbell RL, Li JT, Nicklas RA, et al. Emergency department diagnosis and treatment of anaphylaxis: a practice parameter. Ann Allergy Asthma Immunol 2014;113(6):599–608.
38. Reisman RE, Livingston A. Late-onset allergic reactions, including serum sickness, after insect stings. J Allergy Clin Immunol 1989;84(3):331–7.
39. Peng Z, Simons FE. Advances in mosquito allergy. Curr Opin Allergy Clin Immunol 2007;7(4):350–4.
40. Armentia A, Pineda F, Fernández S. Wine-induced anaphylaxis and sensitization to hymenoptera venom. N Engl J Med 2007;357(7):719–20.
41. Boyle RJ, Elremeli M, Hockenhull J, et al. Venom immunotherapy for preventing allergic reactions to insect stings. Cochrane Database Syst Rev 2012;(10): CD008838.
42. Ruëff F, Vos B, Oude Elberink J, et al. Predictors of clinical effectiveness of Hymenoptera venom immunotherapy. Clin Exp Allergy 2014;44(5):736–46.
43. Cox L, Larenas-Linnemann D, Lockey RF, et al. Speaking the same language: The World Allergy Organization Subcutaneous Immunotherapy Systemic Reaction Grading System. J Allergy Clin Immunol 2010;125(3):569–74, 574.e1–574.e7.

Allergic Dermatoses

Van Nguyen, DO*, Lauren Simon, MD, MPH, Ecler Jaqua, MD

KEYWORDS

- Atopic dermatitis • Contact dermatitis • Urticaria • Angioedema • Eczema

KEY POINTS

- Triggers should be identified and avoided in atopic dermatitis (AD), contact dermatitis (CD), urticaria, and angioedema.
- Pruritus is a required symptom in the diagnosis of AD.
- The mainstay of treatment of AD and CD is topical corticosteroids.
- Urticaria is characterized by superficial tissue swelling, whereas angioedema is deep tissue swelling.
- The preferred treatment of urticaria and angioedema is antihistamines.

INTRODUCTION

The purpose of this article is to review the current available material pertaining to AD, CD, urticaria, and angioedema. This article focuses on the clinical presentation, diagnosis, and management of each of these disorders. Although AD and CD are similar, their development is different and can affect a patient's quality of life. Urticaria and angioedema are also similar, but the differentiation of the two processes is crucial because they have significant morbidity and mortality with different prognoses.

ATOPIC DERMATITIS
Background

AD, also known as atopic eczema, eczema, and dermatitis, is an inflammatory skin condition that affects both children and adults.[1] The condition affects approximately 5% to 20% of people worldwide and 11% of children and 1% to 3% of the adults in the United States.[2–5] The economic burden of AD rivals that of asthma.[6] AD is a pruritic inflammation of the epidermis and dermis that can be acute, subacute, or chronic.[1] It is often associated with a personal or family history of asthma or allergic rhinitis, creating the atopy triad.[1,7]

The authors have nothing to disclose and no conflicts of interest.
Department of Family Medicine, Loma Linda University, 25455 Barton Road, Suite 209B, Loma Linda, CA 92354, USA
* Corresponding author.
E-mail address: vatnguyen@llu.edu

Prim Care Clin Office Pract 43 (2016) 433–449
http://dx.doi.org/10.1016/j.pop.2016.04.011
0095-4543/16/$ – see front matter © 2016 Elsevier Inc. All rights reserved.
primarycare.theclinics.com

The etiology of AD is most likely multifactorial – the result of genetics, pharmacologic abnormalities, skin barrier defects, the environment, and immunologic factors.[5] AD is influenced by environmental factors, such as low humidity and heavily populated, urban areas.[8,9] These environmental factors break down the skin's integrity, triggering an allergen-specific immunoglobulin E (IgE)–mediated hypersensitivity reaction. This hypersensitivity reaction then leads to cytokine dysregulation.[7,9] This immunologic hypothesis, however, is controversial because a majority of children with AD do not demonstrate the presumed IgE-mediated sensitivity to allergens.[10]

Clinical Symptoms and Signs

Depending on age, the clinical symptoms of AD can vary. The infantile stage, up to 2 years of age, is often pruritic, erythematous, and scaly and can have crusted lesions (**Fig. 1**). It may include vesicles and serous exudates. The childhood stage, ages 2 to 12 years, usually has less exudates and may have some evidence of lichenification, presenting as thickened plaques and skin discoloration (**Fig. 2**). The adult stage can present with a chronic and relapsing course, occurs in patients greater than age 12, and is often localized and has evidence of lichenification (**Fig. 3**).[8]

Moreover, the clinical presentation of AD depends on the stage of the disease. Acute and subacute skin lesions are usually intensely pruritic, erythematous papules with evidence of excoriation and serous exudate (**Fig. 4**). Chronic AD still has these papules and excoriations but the skin is also noted to be lichenified.[5]

Pruritus is a required symptom to diagnose AD.[1] It is the intense and constant pruritus that leads to the cycle of itch-scratch-rash-itch. This itch-scratch cycle further disrupts the epidermis and leads to further skin inflammation. This then progresses to the skin lichenification as noted in the childhood and adult stages of AD.[1,8]

Diagnosis

Skin biopsy is of little diagnostic value in the diagnosis of AD.[11,12] Diagnosis of AD is best based on an array of clinical signs and symptoms. In 2003, the American Academy of Dermatology recommended a revised version of the 1980 Hanafin and Rajka and United Kingdom Working Party criteria for AD (**Box 1**). These criteria are preferred to the more extensive 1980 Hanafin and Rajka and United Kingdom Working Party criteria because it can be applied to all age groups.[13]

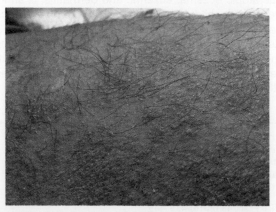

Fig. 1. Atopic dermatitis often consists of erythematous, scaly patches that can be very pruritic.

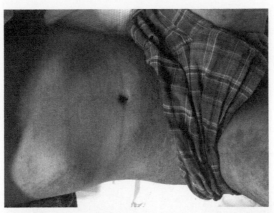

Fig. 2. Chronic atopic dermatitis usually has less exudates and may have thickened plaques, skin discoloration, and evidence of excoriation.

Treatment

AD does not have a cure. Prevention is one of the most important factors in the management plan, but when this cannot be achieved, treatment modalities focuses on alleviating the pruritus and inflammation associated with AD.

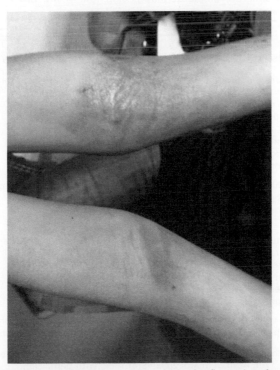

Fig. 3. Classic presentation of atopic dermatitis within the flexural surfaces.

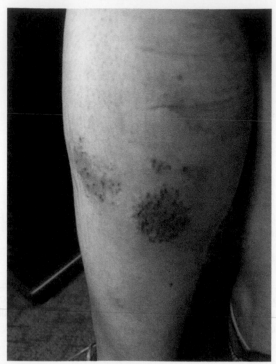

Fig. 4. Acute and subacute atopic dermatitis skin lesions are often intensely pruritic, erythematous patches with papules and serous exudate.

Box 1
Suggested universal criteria for atopic dermatitis by the American Academy of Dermatology

1. Essential features that must be present and, if complete, are sufficient for diagnosis
   a. Pruritus
   b. Eczematous changes that are acute, subacute, or chronic:
      i. Typical and age-specific patterns
         1. Facial, neck, and extensor involvement in infants and children
         2. Current or prior flexural lesions in adults/any age
         3. Sparing of groin and axillary regions
      ii. Chronic or relapsing course

2. Important features that are seen in most cases, adding support to the diagnosis
   a. Early age at onset
   b. Atopy (IgE reactivity)
   c. Xerosis

3. Associated features and clinical associations that may help in the diagnosis of AD
   a. Keratosis pilaris or ichthyosis or palmar hyperlinearity
   b. Atypical vascular responses
   c. Perifollicular accentuation or lichenification or prurigo
   d. Ocular or periorbital changes
   e. Perioral or periauricular lesions

4. The following conditions should be excluded: scabies, allergic CD, seborrheic dermatitis, cutaneous lymphoma, ichthyoses, psoriasis, and other primary disease entities

Adapted from Eichenfield LF, Hanifin JM, Luger TA, et al. Consensus conference on pediatric atopic dermatitis. J Am Acad Dermatol 2003;49(6):1088; with permission.

Emollients/moisturizers
The regular use of emollients can reduce the need for topical corticosteroids and improve symptoms.[14] Emollients should be applied at least twice a day, ideally after a warm-water shower. Patients should be instructed to use nondetergent soap and dry with a soft towel.[9]

Topical corticosteroids
Topical corticosteroids are the mainstay therapy and first-line treatment of AD flares.[15,16] The potency of the topical steroids is classified by its vasoconstrictive properties.[17] Low and moderate potency corticosteroids are preferred on the face, neck, axillae, groin, and flexor surfaces. Steroids are usually applied for 3 to 7 days.[15,18] Lichenified AD, however, may require long-term treatment with high-potency corticosteroids, as noted in **Table 1**.[19]

Once the symptoms have improved, most patients can and should resume emollient use to help prevent flares. In severe cases, long-term maintenance topical corticosteroids are required.[20] Patients need to be warned, however, that long-term use of steroids can cause telangiectasia, striae, hypopigmentation, acne, and even glaucoma if applied near the eyes.[21,22]

Calcineurin inhibitors
Both topical tacrolimus and pimecrolimus are effective in the treatment of AD.[16] These treatments are usually reserved for patients with moderate-to-severe AD that is resistant to corticosteroids or have suffered from steroid-induced skin atrophy.[23] Calcineurin inhibitors are not first-line therapy because the Food and Drug Administration has warned about a possible association of its use with lymphoma, skin cancer, and systemic immunosuppression.[24,25] These associations are still being studied.[26,27]

Antibiotics
Systemic antibiotics help eliminate superimposed infections that can occur with an exacerbation of AD. Staphylococcus aureus is the most common organism and can be treated with short courses of antibiotics, such as floxacillin, cephalexin, or amoxicillin-clavulanate. Topical antibiotics are usually not recommended unless a localized skin infection is present.[28,29]

Antihistamines
The use of oral antihistamines is not generally indicated in the treatment of AD. They may be used, however, for a sedative effect and thus minimize the pruritus and discomfort associated with AD.[9]

Immunosuppressive agents and ultraviolet phototherapy
Widespread AD that is resistant to topical treatment may benefit from ultraviolet phototherapy and immunosuppressive therapy. Therapies, such as systemic corticosteroids, cyclosporine, azathioprine, mycophenolate, and interferon gamma, should be used with the assistance of an experienced dermatologist.[17,30]

Complementary and alternative treatment
Homeopathy, hypnotherapy, biofeedback, and massage therapy do not have good supporting data for the treatment of AD.[15,16] Restrictive diets can lead to malnutrition and thus should not be recommended.[31] Due to the lack of evidence of the benefits of alternative treatment, these modalities should not be recommended for clinical practice.

Table 1			
Relative potencies of topical corticosteroids (relative but not all examples)			
Class	Drug	Dosage Form(s)	Strength (%)
I. Very high potency	Augmented betamethasone dipropionate	Ointment	0.05
	Clobetasol propionate	Cream, foam, ointment	0.05
	Diflorasone diacetate	Ointment	0.05
	Halobetasol propionate	Cream, ointment	0.05
II. High potency	Amcinonide	Cream, lotion, ointment	0.1
	Augmented betamethasone dipropionate	Cream	0.05
	Betamethasone dipropionate	Cream, foam, ointment, solution	0.05
	Desoximetasone	Cream, ointment	0.25
	Desoximetasone	Gel	0.05
	Diflorasone diacetate	Cream	0.05
	Fluocinonide	Cream, gel, ointment, solution	0.05
	Halcinonide	Cream, ointment	0.1
	Mometasone furoate	Ointment	0.1
	Triamcinolone acetonide	Cream, ointment	0.5
III-IV. Medium potencys	Betamethasone valerate	Cream, foam, lotion, ointment	0.1
	Clocortolone pivalate	Cream	0.1
	Desoximetasone	Cream	0.05
	Fluocinolone acetonide	Cream, ointment	0.025
	Flurandrenolide	Cream, ointment	0.05
	Fluticasone propionate	Cream	0.05
	Fluticasone propionate	Ointment	0.005
	Mometasone furoate	Cream	0.1
	Triamcinolone acetonide	Cream, ointment	0.1
V. Lower–medium potency	Hydrocortisone butyrate	Cream, ointment, solution	0.1
	Hydrocortisone probutate	Cream	0.1
	Hydrocortisone valerate	Cream, ointment	0.2
	Prednicarbate	Cream	0.1
VI. Low potency	Alclometasone dipropionate	Cream, ointment	0.05
	Desonide	Cream, gel, foam, ointment	0.05
	Fluocinolone acetonide	Cream, solution	0.01
	Dexamethasone	Cream	0.1
	Hydrocortisone	Cream, lotion, ointment, solution	0.25, 0.5, 1
	Hydrocortisone acetate	Cream, ointment	0.5–1

Adapted from Eichenfield LF, Tom WL, Berger TG, et al. Guidelines of care for the management of atopic dermatitis: Section 2. Management and treatment of atopic dermatitis with topical therapies. J Am Acad Dermatol 2014;71:122; with permission.

Prognosis

The outcome of AD is challenging to predict. More than half of patients suffering from AD have complete resolution of their symptoms.[32,33] Those patients with recurrence of their disease may be predicted by a positive history of early-onset, respiratory disease, such as asthma, atopy, high circulating serum IgE, and a family history of AD.[34] The unpredictable course and unremitting symptoms of AD cause lost work and are at the heart of its economic burden today.[6]

CONTACT DERMATITIS
Background

CD—subacute, acute, and chronic—is caused by an external agent, toxicity, or allergen.[1] In one study, the incidence of CD is 13% to 14%.[35] CD can be divided into 2 categories – allergic and irritant.[36] Allergic CD is less common than irritant CD.[37]

Allergic CD is the classic, delayed-hypersensitivity reaction that can have a latent period of days to years.[1,36] The skin must first be exposed to the foreign substance—physical or chemical irritant—and result in sensitization. The most common causes of allergic CD are poison ivy, nickel, perfumes, dyes, and rubber products.[38] When re-exposed to the foreign substance at a later date, an inflammatory cascade is triggered, the elicitation phase.[36,39]

Irritant CD is not an immune-mediated reaction; it is a nonspecific inflammatory reaction.[1,36,38] It is the result of skin injury from direct contact with an irritant that is of the required concentration and length of exposure.[39] The most common causes of irritant CD are solvents and chemicals that have been in contact with the skin.[38] As such, occupational CD is the most common occupational disease, second to traumatic injury, and thus has a great economic burden on society today.[36]

Clinical Symptoms and Signs

CD can affect any area of the skin, but the hands, face, and neck are most commonly involved.[36] Both allergic and irritant CD share similar symptoms and clinical signs. Both forms of CD can be intensely pruritic.[1,36]

The subacute phase of CD is characterized by mild erythema and small scales or desquamation often associated with small, firm papules.[1] The acute phase of CD has irregular and well-demarcated erythematous and edematous patches, sometimes peppered with vesicles and crusted lesions (**Fig. 5**).[1] The acute phase can last days to weeks.[1,40] Chronic CD can last months to years and is usually characterized by lichenified skin – skin that is thickened, scaly, and fissured and has pigmentation variation (**Figs. 6** and **7**).[1,40]

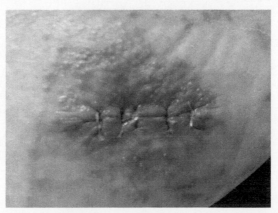

Fig. 5. The acute phase of allergic contact dermatitis has a well-demarcated erythematous and edematous patch, often peppered with vesicles and crusted lesions. This lesion is secondary to neomycin antibiotic ointment application.

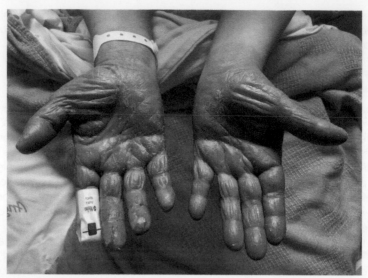

Fig. 6. Chronic irritant contact dermatitis from latex gloves and ritualistic hand-washing with noted erythematous, well-demarcated glove-distribution scales with thickened and fissured digits.

Allergic CD differs from irritant CD in that irritant CD is often associated with burning and pain, whereas allergic CD is predominately pruritic.[36] Moreover, allergic CD usually has distinct angles, lines, and borders, whereas irritant CD has less distinct borders.[41]

Diagnosis

The diagnosis of CD is often based on an accurate history and physical examination and is easier to identify during the acute phase.[39] To differentiate from AD, the arrangement, distribution, and pattern of the skin lesions need to be evaluated. CD

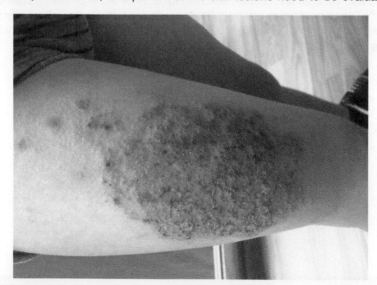

Fig. 7. Subacute irritant contact dermatitis triggered by football pads in a 5-year-old male with noted painful, pruritic, erythematous, scaly, fissured, and thickened skin.

often has an artificial pattern and is isolated to the site of contact (eg, watch dermatitis).[1]

Unfortunately, poor hygiene, neglect, and self-treatment can obscure the diagnosis of CD.[39] In contrast to AD, patch testing may be indicated in CD, especially allergic CD. Positive patch testing has erythema and papules developing after application of the irritant.[1,40]

Treatment

The priority of the treatment of CD is to eliminate the causative factor and initiate preventive measures. Patients should be advised to avoid alkaline soaps, solvents, and detergents. Skin care with emollients and moisturizers should be recommended, including the application of cool compresses, oatmeal baths, and calamine lotion for mild acute vesiculobullous, weeping dermatitis.[38,40]

When prevention cannot be achieved, allergic and irritant CD warrant a similar treatment approach.[40] Topical corticosteroids, applied to presoaked lesions for better penetration and effectiveness, is the mainstay of treatment of these lesions.[42] Localized lesions are treated with high-potency topical corticosteroids and more sensitive areas can be treated with low-potency topical corticosteroids to avoid skin atrophy.[40] Relative potencies of topical steroids are noted in **Table 1**.

When the CD is extensive, involving more than 20% of the skin, however, systemic corticosteroids are usually required.[40] Prednisone 1 mg/kg should be initiated and slowly tapered over 2 to 3 weeks to avoid rebound dermatitis.[38]

Moreover, the use of antibiotics and antihistamines is similar to that of AD. Systemic antibiotic therapy should only be initiated if a secondary infection is noted.[38] Antihistamines are not effective in the treatment of CD but can be used for their sedative effects to minimize nocturnal symptoms to help improve quality of life.[40]

Prognosis

The prognosis is usually good if the offending irritants are removed and preventive measures can be used.[43,44] Negative prognostic factors include disease duration and severity, history of atopy, history of a food-related profession, and remaining in the same profession that has exposed the patient to the known irritant.[45]

URTICARIA
Background

The lifetime prevalence of urticaria, also known as hives, is approximately 20%, without predisposition to age.[42] Urticaria can be induced by physical stimuli, such as cold, pressure, light, heat, exercise, and elevated body temperature.[42,43]

Urticaria has either an immunologic or complement-mediated basis.[1] Immunologic-mediated urticaria results from histamine release from mast cells and is usually in the setting of atopy.[1,44] Complement-mediated urticaria theorizes that anaphylatoxins are released and induce mast-cell degranulation.[1] It is this histamine release that then leads to tissue edema and pruritus, leading to the development of wheals.[42,45]

The etiology of urticaria is vast but it is accepted that the process is provoked by allergens, physical factors, and certain disease processes.[46] Common allergens include foods or food additives (such as strawberries and dyes) and medication exposure, including aspirin, nonsteroidal anti-inflammatory drugs (NSAIDs), and muscle relaxants. Physical factors include cold, pressure, light, heat, exercise, and elevated body temperature. Although rare, certain disease processes, such as Hashimoto disease, can cause urticaria.[42,43]

Clinical Symptoms and Signs

Urticaria are erythematous, raised, circumscribed wheals that blanch with pressure (**Fig. 8**). The wheals range from 1-mm to 2-mm lesions to large 8-cm plaques. Urticaria has no predisposition for body parts; it can be localized or widespread.[42] Patients often report intense pruritus, but some may report flushing and burning.[1,42,47]

The lesions of acute urticarial reactions usually persist 24 hours to 6 weeks. Chronic urticaria can be continuous or intermittent, and, by definition, lasts longer than 6 weeks.[48,49] Usually, no residual symptoms are noted after resolution of the wheals.[42]

Diagnosis

Urticaria is usually a clinical diagnosis, starting with a thorough history and physical, trying to determine the process's cause.[46] Laboratory evaluation of acute urticaria is not recommended unless a specific causes is suspected.[1] Chronic urticaria, on the other hand, should be evaluated with a complete blood cell count, erythrocyte sedimentation rate, and C-reactive protein to evaluate for infection, atopy, and systemic illness. Additionally, further evaluation with thyroid-stimulating hormone level, liver function tests, and urinalysis may help in determining the cause of urticaria.[46] Moreover, patients with a possible specific allergen exposure may also benefit from allergen skin testing.[46]

Treatment

Similar to CD, the most important aspect in the treatment of urticaria is prevention, avoiding known triggers. When prevention is not achieved, a variety of medications can be used to provide patients with relief from their urticaria-associated symptoms.

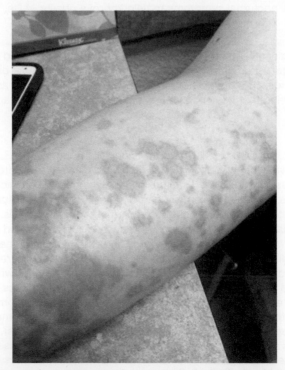

Fig. 8. Urticaria are erythematous, raised, circumscribed wheels that blanch with pressure.

Antihistamines

Second-generation antihistamine drugs, such as fexofenadine, loratadine, desloratadine, cetirizine, and levocetirizine, are the mainstays of treatment of urticaria.[50–52] If symptoms persist longer than 2 weeks, increasing the usual dose of the antihistamine is recommended.[49,53] If still persistent, changing to a different second-generation antihistamine and adding an H_2-blocker, first-generation antihistamine, or leukotriene receptor antagonist may be beneficial.[49,53,54] First-generation antihistamines are helpful in the management of nocturnal symptoms because of their sedative effects.[55] Leukotriene receptor antagonists are especially helpful in patients with cold or NSAID-induced urticaria.[56,57]

Systemic corticosteroids

A short course of systemic corticosteroids should be reserved for severe disease and resistant cases to the first-line and second-line therapy. Small studies suggest that combining systemic corticosteroids and antihistamines can relieve symptoms faster. Due to its potential sequelae, long-term use of corticosteroids is not recommended.[58–60]

Immune modulators

Urticaria that is resistant to the aforementioned treatment modalities may be treated with immunomodulatory therapies under the guidance of a dermatologist. Plasmapheresis and medications, such as cyclosporine, sulfasalazine, hydroxychloroquine, tacrolimus, dapsone, and intravenous immunoglobulin, have been shown beneficial in autoimmune chronic urticaria.[56] Omalizumab, 150 mg or 300 mg every 4 weeks for 3 to 4 cycles, has even been shown to reduce the symptoms and signs of chronic idiopathic urticaria.[61,62]

Prognosis

Approximately half of patients have complete resolution of symptoms within 1 year, but usually, the disease is intermittent and lasts 2 to 5 years.[1,54,63–65] A longer duration of the disease can be predicted by assessing the severity of the disease, presence of thyroid autoimmunology, positive autologous serum skin testing, and any disease complicated by angioedema.[65]

ANGIOEDEMA
Background

Angioedema, regardless of cause, is associated with urticaria in 40% of individuals.[66] The difference between urticaria and angioedema is the depth to which IgE and non-IgE mast cells and basophils are activated.[42,67] Mast cells within the superficial dermis results in urticaria and those in the deeper dermis and subcutaneous tissue result in angioedema.[42] Some forms of angioedema are caused by mediators derived from the bradykinin and complement systems, for example, angiotensin-converting enzyme inhibitor (ACEI)-induced angioedema, which spare the dermis so the angioedema occurs without associated pruritus or hives.

The general term, *angioedema*, is often used to describe a patient's symptoms, but it encompasses several different disease processes with a different pathophysiology. The symptoms of hereditary, C1-inhibitor deficiency, and inherited angioedema are not triggered by an external cause. Hereditary angioedema is an autosomal-dominant disease. On the other hand, allergic angioedema usually has an environmental trigger and is a mast cell–mediated process in 90% of cases. Some cases of angioedema, however, are the result of mostly an IgE-mediated mechanism. This is triggered by similar urticaria allergens – food allergens, such as tree nuts; drug allergens, such as those containing penicillin or sulfa; and environmental allergens, such as fire ants.[68]

Certain medications can also lead to angioedema, including NSAIDs and ACEIs. It is thought that NSAID-associated angioedema is the result of the increased quantity and release of cytokines as triggered by the inhibition of cyclooxygenase 1.[69] ACEI-associated angioedema affects up to 2% of patients using this medication class and is responsible for 30% of cases presenting to emergency departments.[70] It is caused by the inhibition of enzymatic breakdown of tissue bradykinin, causing bradykinin levels to increase.[71] It can occur rapidly or years after introduction of an ACEI.

Clinical Signs and Symptoms

Unlike the widespread effects of urticaria, angioedema often has an abrupt onset with nonpitting, nonpruritic edema of the subcutaneous and submucosal tissues, usually of the face, hands, feet, and trunk.[1,45,68] Angioedema can be, but not always is, accompanied by urticaria.[46] Although less common, angioedema can also effect the abdominal organs, mimicking that of a surgical abdomen, and the fluid shifts within the abdominal cavity can cause hypotension.[45,68] It can even involve the upper airway and cause respiratory compromise.[45]

Hereditary angioedema, unlike acute angioedema, usually has prodromal symptoms and worsens over the first 24 hours and then resolves over the next 3 days. Hereditary angioedema may or may not manifest, anywhere from not once to as frequently as every 3 days.[68]

NSAID-associated angioedema is often associated with urticaria, whereas ACEI-induced angioedema presents without urticaria in approximately 30% of patients.[71] ACEI-induced angioedema commonly presents as face and tongue swelling but can also affect the upper airways and the gastrointestinal tract.[68,71]

Diagnosis

A diagnosis of angioedema starts with a thorough history and physical. It can help distinguish angioedema from other diseases, such as allergic reactions, cellulitis, and acute abdomen.[46]

Once angioedema is diagnosed, allergic angioedema usually responds quickly to treatments (discussed later). Hereditary angioedema can be confirmed by evaluating for C1-inhibitor deficiency.[46] Autoimmune-related angioedema can be evaluated with autologous serum skin testing or in vitro testing of histamine and other mediators.[66] Unfortunately, the cause of chronic angioedema, lasting greater than 6 weeks, is usually unknown.

Treatment

Angioedema treatment is similar to the treatment of urticaria. The most important recommendation is to avoid triggers and control the associated symptoms.[54,72]

Second-generation H_1-receptor antagonists are the preferred treatment to alleviating the symptoms of angioedema.[51,52,73,74] First-generation H_1-receptor blockers can be added to improve nocturnal pruritus. In recalcitrant cases, H_2-receptor antagonists or leukotriene modifiers can be added to the treatment regimen.[54,55,57] Severe cases of angioedema may benefit from a short course of systemic glucocorticoids and even immunomodulatory therapy under the guidance of an experienced dermatologist.[59,60]

Hereditary angioedema, however, can require emergent evaluation and treatment, depending on the site involved. Patients that have angioedema of the larynx may require immediate intubation for airway protection.[75] In such cases, human concentrate C1 inhibitor may be used for acute attacks of hereditary angioedema.[76,77] Fresh-frozen plasma and high-dose 17α-alkylated androgens also can be used as a second-line therapy.[78] Moreover, 17α-alkylated androgens and antifibrinolytic agents can be used to decrease the frequency of these attacks.[79,80] 17α-Alkylated androgens use require regular monitoring of liver enzymes levels and lipids due to the increased liver adenomocarcinoma.[81,82] Antifibrinolytic therapy is dose dependent but can cause muscle cramps and increase the risk for thrombosis.[83,84] Unlike the treatment of urticaria, antihistamines and corticosteroids have not been proved beneficial in the treatment of angioedema.[60]

Prognosis

The prognosis of angioedema is variable because its frequency of attacks cannot be predicted. The frequency of attacks can be reduced with appropriate therapy (discussed previously). Each episode of angioedema, with or without urticaria, can be life threatening. Thus, all measures to identify potential triggers, use prophylactic measures, and preparation for emergency treatment are of the utmost importance.[46] Moreover, due to the high morbidity and mortality, up to 13%, from respiratory compromise associated with angioedema, all patients should be prescribed autoinjectable epinephrine.[85,86]

REFERENCES

1. Wolff K, Johnson R, Suurmond D, et al. Fitzpatrick's color atlas and synopsis of clinical dermatology. New York: McGraw-Hill Medical Pub. Division; 2005.
2. Cury Martins J, Martins C, Aoki V, et al. Topical tacrolimus for atopic dermatitis. Cochrane Database Syst Rev 2015;(7):CD009864.
3. Bath-Hextall FJ, Jenkinson C, Humphreys R, et al. Dietary supplements for established atopic eczema. Cochrane Database Syst Rev 2012;(2):CD005205.
4. Shaw TE, Currie GP, Koudelka CW, et al. Eczema prevalence in the United States: data from the 2003 National Survey of Children's Health. J Invest Dermatol 2011; 131(1):67.
5. Leung DY, Bieber T. Atopic dermatitis. Lancet 2003;361(9352):151–60.
6. Verboom P, hakkaart-Van L, Sturkenboom M, et al. The cost of atopic dermatitis in the Netherlands: an international comparison. Br J Dermatol 2002;147:716–24.
7. Berke R, Singh A, Guralnick M. Atopic dermatitis: an overview. Am Fam Physician 2012;86(1):35–42.
8. Rudikoff D, Lebwohl M. Atopic dermatitis. Lancet 1998;351(9117):1715.
9. Lapidus CS, Honig PJ. Atopic dermatitis. Pediatr Rev 1997;15(8):327–32.
10. Flohr C, Johansson SGO, Wahlgren CF, et al. How atopic is atopic dermatitis? J Allergy Clin Immunol 2004;114:150–8.
11. Hanifin JM, Rajka G. Diagnostic features of atopic dermatitis. Acta Derm Venereol 1980;92(Suppl):44–7.
12. Williams HC. Atopic dermatitis. N Engl J Med 2005;352:2314–24.
13. Eichenfield LF, Tom WL, Berger TG, et al. Guidelines of care for the management of atopic dermatitis: Section 2. Management and treatment of atopic dermatitis with topical therapies. J Am Acad Dermatol 2014;71:116–32.
14. Grimalt R, Mengeaud V, Cambazard F, Study Investigators' Group. The steroid-sparing effect of an emollient therapy in infants with atopic dermatitis: a randomized controlled study. Dermatology 2007;214(1):61–7.

15. National Collaborating Centre for Women's and Children's Health. Atopic eczema in children: management of atopic eczema in children from birth up to the age of 12 years. London (United Kingdom): RCOG Press; 2007. Available at: http://www.nice.org.uk/nicemedia/live/11901/38559/38559.pdf. Accessed January 30, 2012.
16. Hanifin JM, Cooper KD, Ho VC, et al. Guidelines of care of atopic dermatitis, developed in accordance with the American Academy of Dermatology (AAD)/ American Academy of Dermatology Association "Administrative Regulations for Evidence-Based Clinical Practice Guide-lines". J Am Acad Dermatol 2004; 50(3):391–404 [Erratum appears in J Am Acad Dermatol 2005; 52(1):156].
17. McHenry PM, Williams HC, Bingham EA. Management of atopic eczema: Joint Workshop of the British Association of Dermatologists and the Research Unit of the Royal College of Physicians of London. BMJ 1995;310:843–7.
18. Thomas KS, Armstrong S, Avery A, et al. Randomized controlled trial of short bursts of a potent topical corticosteroid versus prolonged use of a mild preparation for children with mild or moderate atopic eczema. BMJ 2002;324:768.
19. Hanifin J, Gupta AK, Rajagopalan R. Intermittent dosing of fluticasone propionate cream for reducing the risk of relapse in atopic dermatitis patients. Br J Dermatol 2002;147:528–37.
20. Berth-Jones J, Damstra RJ, Golsch S, et al. Multinational Study Group. Twice weekly fluticasone propionate added to emollient maintenance treatment to reduce risk of relapse in atopic dermatitis: randomized, double blind, parallel group study. BMJ 2003;326(7403):1367.
21. Werfel T. Topical use of pimecrolimus in atopic dermatitis: update on the safety and efficacy. J Dtsch Dermatol Ges 2009;7(9):739–42.
22. Luger TA, Lahfa M, Folster-Holst R, et al. Long-term safety and tolerability of pimecrolimus cream 1% and topical corticosteroids in adults with moderate to severe atopic dermatitis. J Dermatolog Treat 2004;15:169–78.
23. Berger TG, Duvic M, Van Voorhees AS, et al. The use of topical calcineurin inhibitors in dermatology: safety concerns. Report of the American Academy of Dermatology Association Task Force. J Am Acad Dermatol 2006;54(5):818–23 [Erratum appears in J Am Acad Dermatol 2006;55(2):271].
24. Center for Drug Evaluation and Research. Alert for healthcare professionals: pimecrolimus (marketed as Elidel). Rockville (MD): Food and Drug Administration; 2005. Available at: http://www.fda.gov/cder/drug/InfoSheets/HCP/elidelHCP.htm. Accessed May 9, 2005.
25. Idem. Alert for healthcare professionals: tacrolimus (marketed as Protopic). Rockville (MD): Food and Drug Administration; 2005. Available at: http://www.fda.gov/cder/drug/InfoSheets/HCP/ProtopicHCP.htm. Accessed May 9, 2005.
26. Reitamo S, Wollenberg A, Schöpf E, et al. Safety and efficacy of 1 year of tacrolimus ointment monotherapy in adults with atopic dermatitis. The European Tacrolimus Ointment Study Group. Arch Dermatol 2000;136(8):999–1006.
27. Pariser D. Topical corticosteroids and topical calcineurin inhibitors in the treatment of atopic dermatitis: focus on percutaneous absorption. Am J Ther 2009; 16(3):264–73.
28. Ewing CI, Ashcroft C, Gibbs AC, et al. Flucloxacillin in the treatment of atopic dermatitis. Br J Dermatol 1998;138:1022–9.
29. Suh L, Coffin S, Leckerman KH, et al. Methicillin-resistant Staphylococcus aureus colonization in children with atopic der-matitis. Pediatr Dermatol 2008;25(5): 528–34.
30. Hoare C, Li Wan Po A, Williams H. Systematic review of treatments for atopic eczema. Health Technol Assess 2000;4:1–191.

31. Liu T, Howard RM, Mancini AJ, et al. Kwashiorkor in the United States: fad diets, perceived and true milk allergy, and nutritional ignorance. Arch Dermatol 2001; 137:630–6.
32. Rystedt I. Long term follow-up in atopic dermatitis. Acta Derm Venereol Suppl (Stockh) 1985;114:117–20.
33. Lammintausta K, Kalimo K, Raitala R, et al. Prognosis of atopic dermatitis: a prospective study in early adulthood. Int J Dermatol 1991;30:563–8.
34. Williams HC, Wüthrich B. The natural history of atopic dermatitis. In: Williams HC, editor. Atopic dermatitis: the epidemiology, causes, and prevention of atopic eczema. Cambridge (United Kingdom): Cambridge University Press; 2000. p. 41–59.
35. Mortz CG, Bindslev-Jensen C, Andersen KE. Prevalence, incidence rates and persistence of contact allergy and allergic contact dermatitis in the odense adolescence cohort study: a 15-year follow-up. Br J Dermatol 2013;168(2): 318–25.
36. Usatine RP, Riojas M. Diagnosis and Management of Contact Dermatitis. Am Fam Physician 2010;82(3):249–55.
37. Coenraads PJ. Hand Eczema. N Engl J Med 2012;367:1829–37.
38. Bordel-Gomez MT, Miranda-Romero A, Castrodeza-Sanz J. Epidemiology of contact dermatitis: prevalence of sensitization to different allergens and associated factors. Actas Dermosifiliogr 2010;101(1):59–75.
39. Esterly NB. Contact dermatitis. Pediatr Rev 1979;1(3):85–90.
40. Fonacier L, Bernstein DI, Pacheco K, et al. Contact dermatitis: a practice parameter – update 2015. J Allergy Clin Immunol 2015;3(3 Suppl):S1–39.
41. Usatine RP, Smith M, Mayeaux FJ Jr, et al. Color atlas of family medicine. New York: McGraw-Hill; 2009.
42. Schaefer P. Urticaria: evaluation and treatment. Am Fam Physician 2011;83(9): 1078–84.
43. Grattan CE, Humphreys F. Guidelines for evaluation and management of urticarial in adults and children. Br J Dermatol 2007;157(6):1116–23.
44. Maurer M, Rosen K, Hsieh HJ, et al. Omalizumab for the treatment of chronic idiopathic or spontaneous urticaria. N Engl J Med 2013;368(10):927–35.
45. Muller B. Urticaria and angioedema: a practial appropach. Am Fam Physician 2004;69(5):1123–8.
46. Langley EW, Gigante J. Anaphylaxis, urticaria, and angioedema. Pediatr Rev 2013;34(6):247–56.
47. Fedorowicz Z, van Zuuren EJ, Hu N. Histamine H2-receptor antagonists for urticarial. Cochrane Database Syst Rev 2012;(3):CD008596.
48. Bernstein J, Lang D, Khan D. The diagnosis and management of acute and chronic urticarial: 2014 update. J Allergy Clin Immunol 2014;133(5):1270–7.
49. Powell RJ, Du Toit GL, Siddique N, et al. British Society for Allergy and Clinical Immunology guidelines for the management of chronic urticarial and angioedema. Clin Exp Allergy 2007;37(5):631–50.
50. Sharma M, Bennett C, Cohen SN, et al. H1-antihistamines for chronic spontaneous urticaria. Cochrane Database Syst Rev 2014;(11):CD006137.
51. Charlesworth EN. Urticaria and angioedema: a clinical spectrum. Ann Allergy Asthma Immunol 1996;76(6):454–95.
52. Kennedy MS. Evaluation of chronic eczema and urticarial and angioedema. Immunol Allergy Clin N Am 1999;19(1):19–33.

53. Lin RY, Curry A, Pesola GR, et al. Improved outcomes in patients with acute allergic syndromes who are treated with combined H1 and H2 antagonists. Ann Emerg Med 2000;36(5):462–8.

54. Greaves M. Chronic urticaria. J Allergy Clin Immunol 2000;105(4):664–72.

55. Fox RW. Chronic urticaria: mechanisms and treatment. Allergy Asthma Proc 2001;22(2):97–100.

56. Morgan M, Khan DA. Therapeutic alternatives for chronic urticaria: an evidence-based review, part 1. Ann Allergy Asthma Immunol 2008;100(5):403–11.

57. Ellis MH. Successful treatment of chronic urticarial with leukotriene antagonists. J Allergy Clin Immunol 1998;102(5):876–7.

58. Pollack CV Jr, Romano TJ. Outpatient management of acute urticaria: the role of prednisone. Ann Emerg Med 1995;26(5):547–51.

59. Grattan CE, Sabroe RA, Greaves MW. Chronic urticaria. J Am Acad Dermatol 2002;46:645–57.

60. Blauvelt A, Hwang ST, Udey MC. 11. Allergic and immunologic diseases of the skin. J Allergy Clin Immunol 2003;111(2 suppl):S560–70.

61. Novartis G. Xolair (omalizumab) [package insert]; 2010. Available at: http://www.gene.com/patients/medicines/xolair.

62. Corren J, Casale TB, Lanier B, et al. Safety and tolerability of omalizumab. Clin Exp Allergy 2009;39(6):788–97.

63. Nebiolo F, Bergia R, Bommarito L, et al. Effect of arterial hypertension on chronic urticaria duration. Ann Allergy Asthma Immunol 2009;103:407.

64. Kozel MM, Mekkes JR, Bossuyt PM, et al. Natural course of physical and chronic urticaria and angioedema in 220 patients. J Am Acad Dermatol 2001;45:387.

65. Kulthanan K, Jiamton S, Thumpimukvatana N, et al. Chronic idiopathic urticaria: prevalence and clinical course. J Dermatol 2007;34:294.

66. Kaplan A. Chronic urticaria: pathogenesis and treatment. J Allergy Clin Immunol 2004;114(3):465–74.

67. Carr T, Saltoun C. Urticaria and angioedema. Allergy Asthma Proc 2012;33(1 Suppl):S70–2.

68. Zuraw B. Hereditary angioedema. N Engl J Med 2008;359(10):1027–36.

69. Sanchez-Borges M, Capriles-Hulett A, Caballero-Fonseca F. NSAID-induced urticaria and angioedema: a reappraisal of its clinical management. Am J Clin Dermatol 2002;3(9):599–607.

70. Banerji A, Clark S, Blanda M, et al. Multicenter study of patients with angiotensin-converting enzyme inhibitor-induced angioedema who present to the emergency department. Ann Allergy Asthma Immunol 2008;100:327–32.

71. Kaplan A, Greaves M. Angioedema. J Am Acad Dermatol 2005;53(3):373–88.

72. Joint Task Force on Practice Parameters. The diagnosis and management of urticaria: a practice parameter. Part I: acute urticaria/angioedema. Part II: chronic urticaria/angioedema. Ann Allergy Asthma Immunol 2000;85:521–44.

73. Kaplan AP. Clinical practice: chronic urticaria and angioedema. N Engl J Med 2002;346:175–9.

74. Lee EE, Maibach HI. Treatment of urticaria. An evidence-based evaluation of antihistamines. Am J Clin Dermatol 2001;2:27–32.

75. American College of Allergy, Asthma, & Immunology. Food allergy: a practice parameter. Ann Allergy Asthma Immunol 2006;96(3 Suppl 2):S1–68.

76. Waytes AT, Rosen FS, Frank MM. Treatment of hereditary angioedema with a vapor-heated C1 inhibitor concentrate. N Engl J Med 1996;334:1630–4.

77. Kunschak M, Engl W, Maritsch F, et al. A randomized, controlled trial to study the efficacy and safety of C1 inhibitor concentrate in treating hereditary angioedema. Transfusion 1998;38:540–9.
78. Prematta M, Gibbs JG, Pratt EL, et al. Fresh frozen plasma for the treatment of hereditary angioedema. Ann Allergy Asthma Immunol 2007;98:383–8.
79. Frank MM, Sergent JS, Kane MA, et al. Epsilon aminocaproic acid therapy of hereditary angioneurotic edema: a double-blind study. N Engl J Med 1972;286:808–12.
80. Sheffer AL, Austen KF, Rosen FS. Tranexamic acid therapy in hereditary angioneurotic edema. N Engl J Med 1972;287:452–4.
81. Bork K, Pitton M, Harten P, et al. Hepatocellular adenomas in patients taking danazol for hereditary angioedema. Lancet 1999;353:1066–7.
82. Monnier N, Ponard D, Duponchel C, et al. Characterisation of a new C1 inhibitor mutant in a patient with hepatocellular carcinoma. Mol Immunol 2006;43:2161–8.
83. Cicardi M, Castelli R, Zingale LC, et al. Side effects of long-term prophylaxis with attenuated androgens in hereditary angioedema: comparison of treated and untreated patients. J Allergy Clin Immunol 1997;99:194–6.
84. Bork K, Bygum A, Hardt J. Benefits and risks of danazol in hereditary angioedema: a long-term survey of 118 patients. Ann Allergy Asthma Immunol 2008;100:153–61.
85. Agostoni A, Aygören-Pürsün E, Binkley KE, et al. Hereditary and acquired angioedema: problems and progress: proceedings of the third C1 esterase inhibitor deficiency workshop and beyond. J Allergy Clin Immunol 2004;114:S51.
86. Safdar B, Cone DC, Pham KT. Subcutaneous epinephrine in the prehospital setting. Prehosp Emerg Care 2001;5:200–7.

Indoor and Outdoor Allergies

Madhavi Singh, MD[a],*, Amy Hays, MD[b]

KEYWORDS

- Outdoor allergies • Indoor allergies • Allergens • Pollens • Dust mites
- Mold allergies • Air pollution

KEY POINTS

- In last 30 to 40 years there has been significant increase in the incidence of allergy, likely related to increasing air pollution and changing lifestyles.
- Dust mites, molds, and animal allergens contribute to most of the sensitization in the indoor setting.
- Tree and grass pollens are the leading allergens in the outdoor setting.
- The mainstay of treatment involves avoidance of allergens in many settings, modifying lifestyle, medical treatment, and immunotherapy.

INTRODUCTION

In last 30 to 40 years there has been significant increase in the incidence of allergies. A combination of factors, including genetics, increasing air pollution, and the adoption of modern urbanized lifestyles, has contributed to this increase.[1] The course of allergies is highly variable and the term allergy march is used to describe the natural history of allergic manifestations, including the progression from eczema to asthma that can occur.[2]

An allergen is any substance that elicits an immunoglobulin E (IgE) antibody response. It can be an indoor or outdoor allergen that produces the IgE response, which can manifest as different disease entities, including allergic rhinitis, asthma, allergic conjunctivitis, and contact dermatitis (**Box 1**). Allergic rhinitis and allergic asthma are the most common manifestations of reactions to indoor and outdoor allergens. Allergic rhinitis is characterized by an early type 1 hypersensitivity reaction in an already sensitized person that causes activation of efferent nerve fibers of the respiratory tract and results in rhinorrhea, sneezing, and nasal obstruction.[3] It is estimated

Disclosures: The authors have nothing to disclose.
[a] Department of Family and Community Medicine, Penn State Hershey Medical Group, 1850 East Park Avenue, Suite 207, State College, PA 16803, USA; [b] Department of Family and Community Medicine, Penn State Hershey Medical Group, 303 Benner Pike #1, State College, PA 16803, USA
* Corresponding author.
E-mail address: msingh1@hmc.psu.edu

Prim Care Clin Office Pract 43 (2016) 451–463
http://dx.doi.org/10.1016/j.pop.2016.04.013
0095-4543/16/$ – see front matter © 2016 Elsevier Inc. All rights reserved.

Box 1
Common allergens

Indoor allergens

- Mites
- Animal proteins and animal dander: mites, cats, dogs, cockroaches
- Mold
- Chemicals
- Perfumes
- Pollen
- Smoke

Outdoor allergens

- Pollens: grass, tree, weeds
- Air pollutants
- Mold
- Outdoor animals: horses

---

that 10% to 40% of allergic patients also have asthma, and there is extensive overlap between asthma and allergies.[4–8]

INDOOR ALLERGIES

Many different allergens cause symptoms in an indoor setting (see **Box 1**). The most common ones are mites, dogs, and cats. Pollens, when transported indoors, can cause symptoms.

Mites

House dust mites (HDMs) contribute to an increased prevalence of perennial allergic rhinitis at lower concentrations and asthma at higher concentrations. The main HDM species include *Dermatophagoides farinae*, *Dermatophagoides pteronyssinus*, *Euroglyphus maynei*, and *Blomia tropicalis*. The 2 major HDM allergens are Der f1 and Der p1. Better insulated and more energy-efficient homes can have higher HDM levels, because they result in a warm and humid environment with low ventilation rates that are ideally suited to HDM growth throughout the year.[9]

Mites present in stored products and food matter causing allergic reactions are called storage mites, and are more common in rural areas. They are found mostly in grains such as wheat, corn, oats, and barley; in their byproducts, such as animal food, hay, and straw; and in the dust from the processing facilities and grain storage. Both dust and storage mites are described as domestic mites. They are microscopic. Ideal conditions for their reproduction and development include 75% humidity and a temperature of 15°C (59° Fahrenheit).

The highest concentration of HDMs is found in bedding, especially with increasing temperature and humidity during sleep, and in fabric-covered furniture, soft toys, and carpeting, because these areas harbor their principal food source, which is exfoliated human skin.[10]

Air conditioning plays an important role in gathering HDM allergens.[11]

The initial sensitization from the mites occurs through inhalation, ingestion, or contact with live or dead mites, byproducts of metabolism, or feces, which produce enzymes and proteins that act as allergens.[10] Small particulate matter (PM) in air, with particles less than 2.5 μm in diameter, termed $PM_{2.5}$, have a synergistic effect with mite allergens on coexposure, and cockroach sensitization can mitigate a future allergen response from mites.[12,13]

Animal Allergens

All warm-blooded animals, including birds, are capable of sensitizing susceptible patients but the common manifestation of animal allergy is by domestic dogs and cats. The animal allergens are small proteins produced in the liver or secretory glands and are localized in the animal's skin and body fluids like urine, saliva, blood, milk, and sweat. The allergen proteins adhere to fur and other surfaces and can be efficiently dispersed. They also tend to bind to small dust particles (<10 μm), which can be easily transferred to previously unexposed areas, accumulating in textiles like carpets, upholstered furniture, and mattresses. The indoor concentration of pet allergen depends on factors like lifestyle, carpet versus hard floor, indoor versus outdoor animal, and whether an animal is allowed on a sofa and bed.[14]

The animal allergen causes acute type 1 hypersensitivity symptoms and chronic inflammation of airways that can manifest as allergic rhinitis and asthma. Up to 67% of children with asthma are sensitized to cat and dog allergens and animal allergen exposure results in poor asthma control in sensitized patients.[15]

Although primarily an outdoor allergy exposure for farmers, stable workers, horse riders, and veterinarians, sensitization to horse allergens is more common than expected in urban residents.[15,16] It can induce asthma, urticaria, and eczema despite the low incidence of reported direct contact with horses. The most significant allergen is Equ c1, found in dander and saliva, and to a lesser degree in urine.[17]

Table 1 presents a list of common animal allergens.

Insect Allergens

Debris of many insects has been noted to sensitize and cause allergy responses in the form of allergic rhinitis, asthma, and atopic dermatitis. The most common indoor insect allergen comes from cockroaches. Multiple studies show an association of early exposure of cockroaches and early-onset asthma and allergic rhinoconjunctivitis.[1,18]

Molds and Fungi

Molds proliferate in both indoor and outdoor environments. Ubiquitous contamination by molds is caused by complex interactions of many factors after they enter and colonize the homes via open windows.[19,20] Age and construction of the building, presence

Table 1 Common animal allergen	
Animal	**Common Allergen Protein**
Cat	Fel d1
Dog	Can f1
Mouse	Mus m1
Rat	Rat n1
Horse	Equ c1
Bovine	Bos d2

of a basement or crawl space, the type of heating system, and use of humidifiers and air conditioning influences the concentration of indoor mold.[3,21] Concentrations of airborne fungi are highest in late summer and early autumn, and lowest in winter.[22] Spore counts also vary diurnally, being highest in the afternoon and early evening.

Common molds include *Cladosporium* species, basidiospores, spores of the *Penicillium/Aspergillus* type, and *Alternaria*.[23] Most mold allergens are encountered through inhalation of mold spores.[19] Their spores are heterogeneous in size and shape, varying from 2 to 250 μm, but many are of respirable size. Bronchial and nasal challenge tests have shown that fungal spores or mycelial extracts were both capable of inducing rhinitis or asthma.[24] Threshold concentrations required to trigger allergic reactions are unknown, but increased airborne concentrations of *Alternaria* spores have been associated with a higher risk of respiratory arrest in sensitized patients.[24] Health outcomes are related to concentration of specific fungal genera and not the total or culturable spore counts.[25] Research on fungal allergy is hampered by difficulty in determining the extent of symptoms attributable to fungal exposure, because of coinciding seasons of peak grass and weed pollens.

Most mold-allergic patients are also sensitized to other aeroallergens. The Global Allergy and Asthma European Network found 11.9% sensitization to *Alternaria*, and 5.8% to *Cladosporium herbarum*.[26] Children generally show a higher prevalence of fungal sensitization.

Tobacco Smoke

Increased serum cotinine levels are significantly associated with IgE sensitization to cockroaches, grass pollen, and certain foods, with potential dose-dependent relationships but the association varies for different allergens among children.[27]

Cooking Gas and Nitrogen Dioxide

Weak associations have been noted between short-term nitrogen dioxide (NO_2) exposure from gas cooking and respiratory symptoms and a decrement in lung function parameters in children, but not consistently in exposed women. Children showed increased respiratory symptoms, decreased lung function, and increased incidences of chronic cough, bronchitis, and conjunctivitis with long-term exposure, but adults did not.[28]

Fragrance and Preservatives

Preservative agents, along with fragrance components, are the most important sensitizing agents in cosmetic products and contribute to the most common cause of allergic contact dermatitis.[29] Some terpenes used as fragrance are not allergenic themselves but readily form allergenic products on air exposure.[30] Labeling has been made mandatory by the European Union for 26 fragrance substances commonly known to cause allergic disease.[31,32]

Chemical Allergens

Association with increased risks of respiratory and allergic health effects in children is noted with composite wood materials that emit formaldehyde, flexible plastics that emit plasticizers, and new paint.[33] Propylene glycol and glycol ethers that are present in low concentrations in the bedroom have been noted to be significantly associated with an increased risk of multiple allergic symptoms, asthma, rhinitis, and eczema, and IgE sensitization in preschool-aged children.[34]

Increased humidity in concrete floor constructions and emission of 2-ethyl-1-hexanol, an indicator of dampness-related alkaline degradation of the plasticizer di(ethylhexyl)-phthalate, may be contributing to asthma symptoms.[35]

OUTDOOR ALLERGIES

The source of allergic illness from outdoor allergens can be multiple, with pollens and fungal spores being the primary sources. Particles are released from the sources into the air by wind, rain, mechanical disturbance, or active discharge mechanisms.[36]

Pollens

Pollen allergy affects approximately 40% of individuals with allergies.[37] Pollens are aeroallergens because they are buoyant, water soluble, and produced abundantly. Grass, trees, and weeds are the most common sources of pollen but, in recent decades, ornamental plants provide a new source of aeroallergens. The greatest exposure of pollens is to the upper respiratory tract because of the particle size of 20 to 60µm and thus cause more upper respiratory symptoms. Particles smaller than 3µm are able to penetrate to lung alveoli and contribute to lower respiratory symptoms.[38]

Thunderstorm Asthma

Increased incidence of asthma has been noted at the beginning of thunderstorms during pollen season. During rain and thunderstorms, pollen grains rupture by osmotic shock and release very small (0.5–2 µm) components into the atmosphere that can reach lower airways, inducing asthma reactions in patients with known history of asthma or allergic rhinitis.[39]

Ragweed

Ragweed is one of the most abundant aeroallergens in late summer. It contributes to about half of all cases of pollen-associated allergic rhinitis in North America. Among different types, the short ragweed is the most allergenic weed and the major allergenic compound is identified as Amb a1.

Ragweed allergy usually causes allergic rhinitis and asthma but contact dermatitis has been noted in sensitive individuals. Warmer autumn temperatures and increased carbon dioxide concentration increases ragweed pollen count production and it can extend the growing season for ragweed, thus causing a longer allergy season and higher pollen count.[40,41] Oral allergy syndrome has also been noted in people with ragweed allergy, caused by the cross reactivity of the allergen found in ragweed with those in some fruits and vegetables, such as banana, melon, chamomile, watermelon, cucumber, and zucchini.

Grass

Grass pollens contain 20 to 40 different antigens, which have been categorized into 8 groups, based on their immunologic characteristics. Allergens of group I, averaging 3 µm in diameter, are extracted from the outer wall of pollen grains and starch granules.[42] The importance of this group is shown by the fact that 90% to 95% of patients who are grass pollen allergic react to group I allergens on skin testing. Groups II and III cause reactions in 60% to 70% of these patients.[43] Much less is known about the remaining 8 groups of grass pollens. Grass pollens as aeroallergens play a role in pathogenesis of atopic dermatitis in children.[44]

Tree Pollen

Tree pollen allergies are mainly elicited by allergenic trees belonging to the orders Fagales, Lamiales, Proteales, and Pinales. The major birch pollen allergen Bet v1 gene was the first gene to be cloned, and since then, 53 tree pollen allergens have been identified and acknowledged.[37] Because a high degree of cross-sensitization exists among tree pollens, testing with birch pollen allergen is sufficient for the diagnostic screening of tree pollen allergy.[45] Bet v1 cross reacts with low-molecular-weight apple allergen, causing an association with oral apple sensitivity. This same cross reactivity applies to pear, celery, carrot, and potato allergens.[46] In Japan, the Japanese cedar is the most significant tree allergen, whereas olive tree pollen is important in Mediterranean regions.

AIR POLLUTANTS

Air pollutants in the form of PM are mixtures of solid and liquid particles suspended in air. There are other gases and chemicals that contribute to air pollutants. Coal and oil fuel combustion for construction and agricultural operations, power plants, industries, heating, cooking, and lighting produce these ubiquitous particles, with more than 80% attributed to diesel exhaust.[1,47] These sources contribute to PM and pollutants.

Particulate Matter and Pollutants

A mixture of solid and liquid particles suspended in air, PM can have different sizes, shapes, and chemical composition[1] (Fig. 1). The size of PM and pollutants determines the level of penetration in the airway and the resulting illness.[47] They can be transported over long distances and their removal may occur via rainfall, gravitational sedimentation, or coagulation with other particles.[1]

The World Health Organization 2005 Air Quality Standards set goals for daily exposure to less than 25 $\mu g/m^3$ for $PM_{2.5}$ and less than 50 $\mu g/m^3$ for PM_{10}.[47] Pollution from

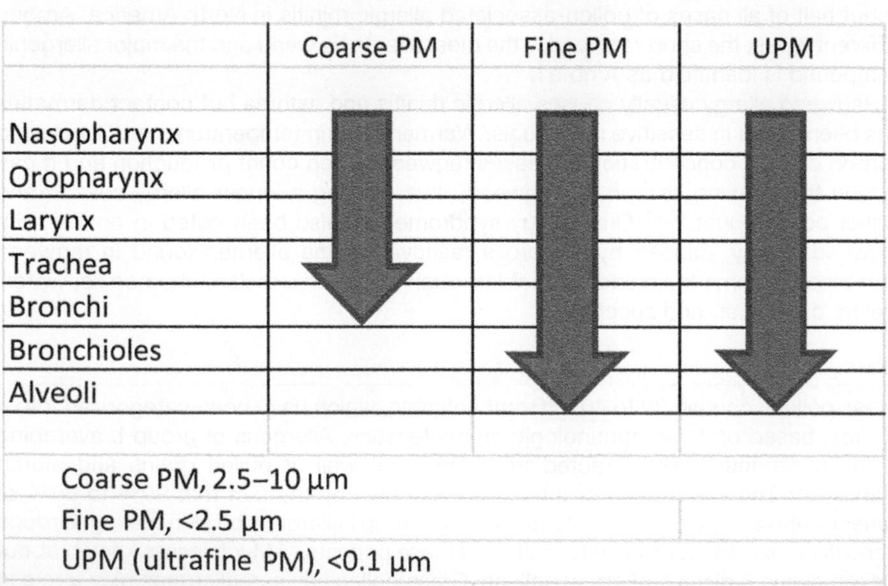

	Coarse PM	Fine PM	UPM
Nasopharynx			
Oropharynx			
Larynx			
Trachea			
Bronchi			
Bronchioles			
Alveoli			
Coarse PM, 2.5–10 μm			
Fine PM, <2.5 μm			
UPM (ultrafine PM), <0.1 μm			

Fig. 1. Penetration of PM into the respiratory system.

PM in urban areas often far exceeds this level. Also, there is no evidence of a safe level of exposure.[1] Multiple studies worldwide have shown an association of PM exposure and asthma, allergic rhinitis, and pollen sensitization. No association has been noted with atopic dermatitis.[1] Increased allergic symptoms, reduced lung function, and increased sensitization to common aeroallergens is noted in those living in close proximity to roads (about 100 m) and high traffic density.[1] Studies have shown that diesel exhaust particles can act as mucosal adjuvants and can induce allergic sensitization to a neoallergen in human mucosa.[48]

See **Box 2** for an outline of the composition, source, and formation of PM and pollutants.

DIAGNOSIS

Apart from history and clinical findings, skin testing and/or specific IgE serologic measurements to identify IgE-mediated sensitization is required. Skin testing is the mainstay of diagnosis except for challenges with mold allergen because of a lack of consistent standardized extract. In vitro tests are acceptable substitutes for skin tests in some circumstances, such as in patients with history of anaphylaxis, or in combative or mentally challenged adults. Positive tests for allergen-specific IgE do not diagnose allergy.[49] When there is concern of perennial allergic rhinitis and the patient's history is inconclusive, nasal provocative testing is indicated.[10]

TREATMENT

Lifestyle modification through multiple interventions is often helpful (**Box 3, Tables 2 and 3**).[50–57]

Medication Treatment

Medication for asthma management is mainly based on inhaled corticosteroid and bronchodilator, with varying frequency depending on the severity of symptoms (**Box 4**).

Box 2
Composition, source, and formation of PM and pollutants

Primary PM

Primary PM is directly derived from human and natural activities.

Secondary PM

Formed in the atmosphere from the gaseous precursors emitted in the air. The gaseous precursors are sulfur dioxide (SO_2), oxides of nitrogen (NO_x), ammonia (NH_3) and nonmethane volatile organic compounds.

Primary pollutants

Come from human/natural activity sources: carbon monoxide, nitrogen dioxide (NO_2), SO_2, and polycyclic aromatic hydrocarbons.

Secondary pollutants

Formed in the atmosphere: ozone formed by reaction between NO_2 and volatile organic compounds in the presence of heat and sunlight.

Box 3
Lifestyle modification/in-house air filtration

Whole-house filtration (WHF)

- WHF via a heating, ventilation, air conditioning system is only useful if high-efficiency filters are used. The inexpensive, low-efficiency filters do not offer any particle removal.

High-efficiency particulate air (HEPA) portable room air cleaners (PRACs)

- HEPA PRAC effectiveness is limited to a single room. Multiple units need to be used for different rooms to get the benefit.

Breathing zone filtration

- HEPA sleep breathing zone filtration designed to clean the breathing zone has been shown to be very effective in particle removal.

Combination filtration

- Combination filtration using high-efficiency WHF with PRAC or breathing zone filtration in the bedroom may be the best and most cost-effective approach.

Ionic electrostatic room air cleaner

- Ionic electrostatic room air cleaners provide no benefit compared with the WHF or HEPA PRACs.

Data from Sublett JL. Effectiveness of air filters and air cleaners in allergic respiratory diseases: a review of the recent literature. Curr Allergy Asthma Rep 2011;11(5):395–402.

Table 2
Lifestyle modifications for dust mites, animal allergens, and pollen

Dust Mites	
Avoiding allergen[50]	• Frequent dusting and vacuuming along with weekly washing of bedding in hot water ≥50°C • Physical barriers in the form of allergen-proof encasings for mattresses, pillows, box springs, and bedding • Plastic, wood, or leather furniture instead of upholstered furniture • Replacing carpeting with wood or vinyl flooring • Remove stuffed animals from affected child's room[50]
Low relative humidity	Low humidity inside the house hinders the proliferation of the mites[50,51]
Chemicals	• Acaricides lead to an elimination of 65%–100% of the mites in a mite culture and has shown improvement of asthma and rhinitis • Tannic acid, which is a protein-denaturing agent, can reduce the allergenicity of the house dust[50]
Animal Allergen	
Avoiding allergen	• Removing the offending animal from the house • Animal washing on twice-weekly basis to bring the allergen counts down[52] • Keeping animals out of bedroom
Pollens	
Avoiding allergen	• Staying indoor during high pollen counts • Nasal air filters have been found to be effective in preventive role for managing seasonal allergic rhinitis[53]

Data from Refs.[50–53]

Table 3
Lifestyle modifications for fungi, air pollution, and other allergens

Fungus

Indoor mold control	• Fungicide can be used to control mold in the air conditioner • Careful cleaning of humidifiers and vaporizers • Placement of a plastic vapor barrier over exposed soil in crawl spaces • Dehumidifiers used in basements and other damp areas may help reduce mold levels[14]

Air Pollution

Limiting exposure	• Heeding smog alerts • Avoiding outdoor exercise • Avoid driving with car windows down[54]

Miscellaneous

Polyphenols	Oral ingestion of apple polyphenols found in unripe apples are found to be effective in alleviating symptoms of persistent allergic rhinitis[55]
In-home test kit to assess allergen level	Use of in-home test kits to regularly assess the allergen level and thus changing behavior and attitude to reduce dust mite allergen levels is also beneficial[56]
Quitting smoking	Those around the allergic person all the time should be encouraged to quit smoking
Preventive measure for allergy march	Probiotics, exclusive breastfeeding or hydrolyzed formula, and immunotherapy for inhalant allergen[2]

Data from Refs.[2,14,54–56]

Box 4
Allergic rhinitis treatment

Mild intermittent symptoms

Oral antihistamines

Intranasal antihistamines

Decongestants

LTRA

Moderate intermittent or mild persistent symptoms

All above, and may add:
  Intranasal corticosteroids
  LTRA

Moderate or severe persistent symptoms

All above; if improved, consider step-down treatment

If not improved, consider infection, noncompliance, or other causes

Can increase dose of intranasal steroid, add ipratropium or oral steroid

Consider referral to specialist

Abbreviation: LTRA, leukotriene receptor antagonists.

IMMUNOTHERAPY

Allergen-specific immunotherapy offers more definitive treatment. Immunotherapy can be recommended when symptoms have already been present for at least 2 years and allergen avoidance is either impossible or insufficient.

Immunotherapy is usually recommended for between 3 and 5 years. In cases of seasonal allergens, such as pollens, updosing is usually started and completed well in advance of the specific pollen season to avoid initiating the treatment of allergic patients with ongoing symptoms and hence to minimize the risk of side effects.[40]

In cases of mold allergy, asthma has long been considered to be a contraindication for immunotherapy. However, molecular cloning helps to enable the development of vaccines for *Alternaria* and other fungi.[23] In 2014, the US Food and Drug Administration approved 3 types of under-the-tongue tablets to treat allergies to grass and ragweed.

SUMMARY

The significant increase in the incidence of allergy in last few decades cannot be explained by genetic factors alone. Increasing air pollution and its interaction with biological allergens, along with changing lifestyles, are contributing factors. Dust mites, molds and animal allergens contribute to most of the sensitization in the indoor setting. Tree and grass pollens are the leading allergens in the outdoor setting. Worsening air pollution and increasing quantities of PM worsen the allergy symptoms and associated morbidity. Cross-sensitization of one allergen to many other allergens is common. The mainstay of treatment involves avoidance of allergens in many settings, modifying lifestyle, medical treatment, and immunotherapy.

REFERENCES

1. Baldacci S, Maio S, Cerrai S, et al. Allergy and asthma: effects of the exposure to particulate matter and biological allergens. Respir Med 2015;109:1089–104.
2. Gordon BR. The allergic march: can we prevent allergies and asthma? Otolaryngol Clin North Am 2011;44(3):765–77.
3. Gerth van Wijk RG, de Graaf-in't Veld C, Garrelds IM. Nasal hyperreactivity. Rhinology 1999;37:50–5.
4. Min YG, Choi BY, Kwon SK, et al. Multicenter study on the prevalence of perennial allergic rhinitis and allergy-associated disorders. J Korean Med Sci 2001;16: 697–701.
5. Linneberg A, Nielsen H, Frolund L, et al. The link between allergic rhinitis and allergic asthma: A prospective population-based study. The Copenhagen Allergy Study. Allergy 2002;57:1048–52.
6. Bousquet J, Annesi-Maesano I, Carat F, et al. Characteristics of intermittent and persistent allergic rhinitis: DREAMS study group. Clin Exp Allergy 2005;35: 728–32.
7. Leynaert B, Neukirch C, Kony S, et al. Association between asthma and rhinitis according to atopic sensitization in a population-based study. J Allergy Clin Immunol 2004;113:86–93.
8. Downie SR, Anderson M, Rimmer J, et al. Association between nasal and bronchial symptoms in subjects with persistent allergic rhinitis. Allergy 2004;59:320–6.
9. Zheng YW, Li J, Lai XX, et al. Allergen micro-array detection of specific IgE- reactivity in Chinese allergy patients. Chin Med J (Engl) 2011;124:4350–4.

10. Vogel P, Morelo Dal Bosco S, Juarez Ferla N. Mites and the implications on human health. Nutr Hosp 2015;31(2):944–51.
11. Zhan X, Li C, Xu H, et al. Air-conditioner filters enriching dust mites allergen. Int J Clin Exp Med 2015;8(3):4539–44.
12. Wang IJ, Tung TH, Tang CS, et al. Allergens, air pollutants, and childhood allergic diseases. Int J Hyg Environ Health 2016;219(1):66–712.
13. He W, Jimenez F, Martinez H, et al. Cockroach sensitization mitigates allergic rhinoconjunctivitis symptom severity in patients allergic to house dust mites and pollen. J Allergy Clin Immunol 2015;136(3):658–66.
14. Zahradnik E, Raulf M. Animal allergens and their presence in the environment. Front Immunol 2014;5:76.
15. Cavkaytar O, Soyer O, Şekerel BE. A rare cause of aeroallergen-induced anaphylaxis: horse allergy. Turk J Pediatr 2014;56:437–9.
16. Liccardi G, D'Amato G, Antonicelli L, et al. Sensitization to horse allergens in Italy: a multicenter study in urban atopic subjects without occupational exposure. Int Arch Allergy Immunol 2011;155(4):412–71.
17. Kim JL, Elfman L, Mi Y, et al. Current asthma and respiratory symptoms among pupils in relation to dietary factors and allergen in the school environment. Indoor Air 2005;15(3):170–82.
18. Donohue KM, Al-alem U, Perzanowski MS, et al. Anti-cockroach and anti-mouse IgE are associated with early wheeze and atopy in an inner-city birth cohort. J Allergy Clin Immunol 2008;122(5):914–20.
19. Dallongeville A, Le Cann P, Zmirou-Navier D, et al. Concentration and determinants of molds and allergens in indoor air and house dust of French dwellings. Sci Total Environ 2015;536:964–72.
20. Sakiyan N, Inceoglu O. Atmospheric concentrations of Cladosporium Link and Alternaria Nees spores in Ankara and the effects of meteorologic factors. Turk J Bot 2003;27:77–81.
21. Wilson SC, Palmatier RN, Andriychuk LA, et al. Mold contamination and air handling units. J Occup Environ Hyg 2007;4(7):483–91.
22. Green BJ, Yli-Panula E, Tovey ER. Halogen immunoassay, a new method for the detection of sensitization to fungal allergens; comparisons with conventional techniques. Allergol Int 2006;55:131–9.
23. Twaroch TE, Curin M, Valenta R, et al. Mold allergens in respiratory allergy: from structure to therapy. Allergy Asthma Immunol Res 2015;7(3):205–20.
24. Licorish K, Novey HS, Kozak P, et al. Role of Alternaria and Penicillium spores in the pathogenesis of asthma. J Allergy Clin Immunol 1985;76:819–25.
25. Osborne M, Reponen T, Adhikari A, et al. Specific fungal exposures, allergic sensitization, and rhinitis in infants. Pediatr Allergy Immunol 2006;17(6):450–7.
26. Heinzerling L, Frew AJ, Bindslev-Jensen C, et al. Standard skin prick testing and sensitization to inhalant allergens across Europe – A study from the GALEN network. Allergy 2005;60:1287–300.
27. Yao TC, Chang SW, Hua MC, et al. Tobacco smoke exposure and multiplexed immunoglobulin E sensitization in children: a population-based study. Allergy 2016;71(1):90–8.
28. Schwela D. Air pollution and health in urban areas. Rev Environ Health 2000; 15(1–2):13–42.
29. Nardelli A, Drieghe J, Claes L, et al. Fragrance allergens in 'specific' cosmetic products. Contact Dermatitis 2011;64(4):212–9.
30. Matura M, Sköld M, Börje A, et al. Selected oxidized fragrance terpenes are common contact allergens. Contact Dermatitis 2005;52(6):320–8.

31. Leijs H, Broekhans J, van Pelt L, et al. Quantitative analysis of the 26 allergens for cosmetic labeling in fragrance raw materials and perfume oils. J Agric Food Chem 2005;53(14):5487–91.
32. Mann J, McFadden JP, White JM, et al. Baseline series fragrance markers fail to predict contact allergy. Contact Dermatitis 2014;70(5):276–81.
33. Mendell MJ. Indoor residential chemical emissions as risk factors for respiratory and allergic effects in children: a review. Indoor Air 2007;17(4):259–77.
34. Choi H, Schmidbauer N, Sundell J, et al. Common household chemicals and the allergy risks in pre-school age children. PLoS One 2010;5(10):e13423.
35. Norbäck D, Wieslander G, Nordström K, et al. Asthma symptoms in relation to measured building dampness in upper concrete floor construction, and 2-ethyl-1-hexanol in indoor air. Int J Tuberc Lung Dis 2000;4(11):1016–25.
36. Burge HA, Rogers CA. Outdoor allergens. Environ Health Perspect 2000;108(Suppl 4):653–9.
37. Asam C, Hofer H, Wolf M, et al. Tree pollen allergens-an update from a molecular perspective. Allergy 2015;70(10):1201–11.
38. Platts-Mills TAE. The allergy epidemics: 1870-2010. J Allergy Clin Immunol 2015;136(1):3–13.
39. D'Amato G, Liccardi G, Frenguelli G. Thunderstorm-asthma and pollen allergy. Allergy 2007;62(1):11–6.
40. El-Qutob D. Vaccine development and new attempts of treatment for ragweed allergy. Ther Adv Vaccines 2015;3(2):41–7.
41. Enberg RN, Leickly FE, McCullough J, et al. Watermelon and ragweed share allergens. J Allergy Clin Immunol 1987;79(6):867–75.
42. Ford SA, Baldo BA. A re-examination of rye grass (Lolium perenne) pollen allergens. Int Arch Allergy Appl Immunol 1986;81:193–203.
43. Staff IA, Taylor PE, Smith P, et al. Cellular localization of water soluble, allergenic proteins in ryegrass pollen using monoclonal & specific IgE antibodies with immunogold probes. Histochem J 1990;22:276–90.
44. Sybilski AJ, Zalewska M, Furmańczyk K, et al. The prevalence of sensitization to inhalant allergens in children with atopic dermatitis. Allergy Asthma Proc 2015;36(5):81–5.
45. Eriksson NE, Wihl JA, Arrendal H, et al. Tree pollen allergy. II. Sensitization to various tree pollen allergens in Sweden. A multi-centre study. Allergy 1984;39(8):610–7.
46. Valenta R, Duchene M, Vrtalas S, et al. Recombinant allergens for immunoblot diagnosis of tree-pollen allergy. J Allergy Clin Immunol 1991;88:889–94.
47. Huang S-K, Zhang Q, Qiu Z, et al. Mechanistic impact of outdoor air pollution on asthma & allergic diseases. J Thorac Dis 2015;7(1):23–33.
48. Diaz-Sanchez D, Garcia MP, Wang M, et al. Nasal challenge with diesel exhaust particles can induce sensitization to a neoallergen in the human mucosa. J Allergy Clin Immunol 1999;104:1183–8.
49. Ownby DR. Allergy testing: in vivo versus in vitro. Pediatr Clin North Am 1988;35(5):995–1009.
50. Pauli G, Bessot JC, Dietemann-Molard A, et al. Prevention of asthma caused by dust mites. Rev Mal Respir 1993;10(1):1–7.
51. Moungthong G, Klamkam P, Mahakit P, et al. Efficacy of the Precise Climate Controller on the reduction of indoor microorganisms. Asia Pac Allergy 2014;4(2):113–8.

52. Hodson T, Custovic A, Simpson A, et al. Washing the dog reduces dog allergen levels, but the dog needs to be washed twice a week. J Allergy Clin Immunol 1999;103(4):581–5.
53. Kenney P, Hilberg O, Laursen AC, et al. Preventive effect of nasal filters on allergic rhinitis: a randomized, double-blind, placebo-controlled crossover park study. J Allergy Clin Immunol 2015;136(6):1566–72.e1-5.
54. Guarnieri M, Balmes JR. Outdoor air pollution & asthma. Lancet 2014;383: 1581–92.
55. Enomoto T, Nagasako-Akazome Y, Kanda T, et al. Clinical effects of apple polyphenols on persistent allergic rhinitis: a randomized double-blind placebo-controlled parallel arm study. J Investig Allergol Clin Immunol 2006;16(5):283–9.
56. Winn AK, Päivi M, Klein C, et al. Efficacy of an in-home test kit in reducing dust mite allergen levels: results of a randomized controlled pilot study. J Asthma 2015;26:1–6.
57. Sublett JL. Effectiveness of air filters and air cleaners in allergic respiratory diseases: a review of the recent literature. Curr Allergy Asthma Rep 2011;11(5): 395–402.

Allergic Rhinitis

Hasan A. Kakli, MD*, Timothy D. Riley, MD

KEYWORDS

- Allergic rhinitis • Type 1 hypersensitivity • Vasomotor rhinitis • Skin prick testing
- Serum-specific Ig E • Allergen immunotherapy • Chronic rhinosinusitis
- Nasal polyps

KEY POINTS

- Allergic rhinitis affects up to 1 in 6 individuals, with health care costs estimated in the billions of dollars.
- Allergic rhinitis is a type 1 IgE-mediated hypersensitivity reaction and usually presents with typical symptomatology.
- Allergic rhinitis can be diagnosed by history and physical examination, with testing reserved for treatment of nonresponders or when identification of the specific cause is necessary to guide treatment.
- There are many therapeutic options, with intranasal corticosteroids the single most effective agent.

INTRODUCTION

Rhinitis is defined as inflammation of the nasal mucosa and affects up to 40% of the population. Among all causes of mucosal inflammation, allergic rhinitis (AR) is the most common, affecting 1 in 6 individuals. Symptoms of AR interfere with all facets of daily life and are associated with reduced quality of sleep and work performance.[1] Previously thought of as a disease restricted to the nasal passages, AR is now viewed as a manifestation of systemic airway disease and is often comorbid in patients with asthma. As a type 1 IgE-mediated hypersensitivity process, symptoms of AR are triggered by allergens; thus, minimizing allergen exposure should be an essential component of any treatment plan. AR often goes undetected by clinicians due to its nature as a long-standing condition. Patients suffering from AR may not seek medical treatment because they often fail to recognize its impact on their daily lives. As such, physicians should routinely screen for this widespread and debilitating condition with a focused history and physical examination.

EPIDEMIOLOGY

Approximately 10% to 20% of the global population suffers from AR, the most common cause of reversible nasal congestion. The reported prevalence of AR has

Penn State Milton S. Hershey Medical Center, Department of Family & Community Medicine, 500 University Drive, Hershey, PA 17033, USA
* Corresponding author.
E-mail address: hkakli@hmc.psu.edu

Prim Care Clin Office Pract 43 (2016) 465–475
http://dx.doi.org/10.1016/j.pop.2016.04.009
0095-4543/16/$ – see front matter © 2016 Elsevier Inc. All rights reserved.

been steadily increasing. The true incidence likely remains underestimated, however, because data collection hinges on physician diagnosis and misses those who are undiagnosed or self-medicate. In the United States, AR is the most common atopic condition, affecting between 9% and 16% of the population. Of patients with AR, 80% develop symptoms before the age of 20.[2] Further highlighting the significance of AR in the pediatric population, in the United States from 1994 to 2002, the prevalence of AR in more than 2000 children ages 13 to 14 years increased from 13% to 19%.[3]

The direct health-related cost expenditure of AR is estimated to be between $2 billion and $5 billion per year with an additional $2 billion to $4 billion lost in annual productivity.[4] A 2007 cohort of more than 8000 US workers revealed that AR caused greater loss of productivity than any other illness, including hypertension, diabetes, and heart disease, and accounted for approximately one-quarter of all lost productivity.[5] In 2006, AR accounted for more than 12 million office visits in the United States, making it the 16th most common primary diagnosis for outpatient office visits.[4] The prevalence and burden of AR obligates primary care providers to be able to readily and cost-effectively diagnose and manage this chronic condition.

CLINICAL PRESENTATION

The clinical presentation of AR is a consequence of its pathophysiology as a classic allergen response. Inflammatory mediators, including mast cells, macrophages, eosinophils, and lymphocytes, enter the nasal mucosa after introduction of the inciting allergen. The most common allergens include dust mite fecal particles, animal dander, molds, and pollens.[6] Identification of the inciting agent is not always necessary to effectively treat AR.

The structure and histology of the nose is designed to allow it to function as a wet filter. Its main purpose is to humidify inhaled air. To accomplish this, the nose must maintain an extensive vascular network allowing it to produce copious amount of mucous, which in the average adult nose averages 2 cups of mucous daily.[7] The mucous captures inhaled particles, gases, and vapors at which point ciliated cells direct them to the back of the throat, allowing them to be swallowed thus diverting them from the lower respiratory tract.[8] This postnasal drip is actually a normal physiologic process. Its consequences, however, such as pharyngitis, vocal cord dysfunction, and cough, indicate potential pathology.[7] When the captured particles incite the IgE-mediated allergy cascade, symptoms soon follow.

As a mucosal antibody, IgE is found in the lining of the eyes, nose, and lower airways. Basophils and mast cells are activated when an allergen bridges 2 specific IgE molecules. The principal vasoactive elements, including histamine, leukotrienes, and prostaglandins, are responsible for the initial phase of symptoms. Inflammatory cells, such as eosinophils, macrophages, and neutrophils, are then recruited, and their arrival leads to further release of vasoactive mediators, producing a delayed-phase inflammatory response. This second wave of symptoms occurs 4 to 6 hours after exposure to the inciting allergen.[9]

The classic symptoms of AR are nasal congestion, nasal itching, sneezing, and rhinorrhea. Allergic conjunctivitis presents as itchy, watery eyes resulting from the same pathophysiology as AR and is not surprisingly a common comorbid condition. Patients may not attribute their symptoms to seasonality or surrounding environments and present with what they believe to be a viral-related illness. Patients' degrees of atopy vary from minimal to severe and symptoms of AR exhibit a similar pattern. For many patients, AR-induced nasal congestion is not merely a trivial stuffy nose but a debilitating problem. A 2007 prospective, cross-sectional survey, identifying symptom perception among patients and providers, revealed that AR-related symptoms had a significant impact on work or school performance in 74% of patients. Sleep patterns were affected for approximately 50% of patients, whereas 61% of patients reported feeling tired, 38% reported feeling irritable, and 23.5% reported a general malaise.[10]

Clinical manifestations depend heavily on age of presentation. Adults and older children suffering from rhinorrhea report blowing their noses constantly during the day. Younger children who have not yet learned this technique will snort, sniff, or cough in an effort to expel secretions. Some children may demonstrate an audible palatal click as the tongue scratches the hard palate. Repeated manipulation or rubbing of the nose due to persistent congestion or drainage can cause excoriations of the external nares and a permanent crease at the juncture of the middle and lower thirds of the nasal bridge.[11] Due to the constant inflammation and subsequent increase in blood flow, venous engorgement in the periorbital region may produce allergic shiners. Other manifestations in the head involve changes consistent with allergic facies seen in children as a consequence of mouth breathing from nasal obstruction: open mouth with receding chin and overbite, elongation of the face, and high arching palate.[9]

As an allergen-mediated disorder of the nasal passage, AR shares several similarities with another allergic disease of the lower respiratory tract: asthma. Not surprisingly, the 2 conditions are often comorbid; 85% of patients with asthma have AR whereas 40% of patients suffering from AR have or will develop asthma. Consequently, the Allergic Rhinitis and its Impact in Asthma guidelines recommend evaluating patients with one condition for the presence of the other.[12] It is now widely accepted that the upper and lower airways represent a continuum of the respiratory tract because they share several physiologic and morphologic features. Allergen cross-linking of IgE receptors results in nasal obstruction in the heavily vascularized nasal passage whereas the same process produces bronchoconstriction in the smooth muscle lined bronchi. AR may promote or exacerbate asthma via different mechanisms. Excessive postnasal drip irritates the lower respiratory tract while the preferential mouth breathing allows cold, dry air to enter the lungs and potentiate bronchial hyper-reactivity. In addition to this, the rhinobronchial reflex, a vagal-mediated response, can cause bronchial constriction as a result of nasal stimulation.[12]

It is important to distinguish AR from other forms of nasal inflammation, namely non-AR. Non-AR can be classified into 9 subtypes, including infectious, gustatory, vasomotor, drug induced, and hormone induced. Hormonal-induced rhinitis includes pregnancy-related rhinitis that can affect 20% to 30% of pregnancies at any gestational age[13] and usually resolves spontaneously within 2 weeks of delivery.[14]

Vasomotor rhinitis (VMR), also known as idiopathic rhinitis, compromises the majority of non-AR causes.[14] The pathophysiology of VMR is poorly understood and may involve increased cholinergic activity, dysfunctional nociceptive receptors that are stimulated in response to innocuous stimuli.[15] Environmental factors trigger symptoms and common causes include inhalation of cold air, changes in temperature, humidity, or barometric pressure, and even strong emotions. Typical symptoms of VMR are rhinorrhea, congestion, postnasal drip, headaches, throat clearing, and coughing. Sneezing and nasal itching are generally mild or absent, a key differentiating feature between VMR and AR. Ocular symptoms also tend to be minimal in VMR because the dysfunction is confined to the nasal mucosa and not representative of an underlying allergy-mediated response.[14]

It is important to remember that many symptoms involving the nose or nasal passages may be due to other disease states and the red flag symptoms, discussed later, should prompt clinicians to seek an alternate diagnosis: unilateral obstruction with or without pain, recurrent epistaxis, mucopurulent rhinorrhea, or anosmia.[11]

DIAGNOSIS

A history marked by typical allergy symptoms forms the basis for diagnosing AR. The diagnosis is likely when 2 or more of the classic AR symptoms of nasal congestion, rhinorrhea, sneezing, and itching are present for more than 1 hour on most days.[16]

Clinicians should try to identify a patient's allergic trigger through the history. Common allergens that should be evaluated for include pollen, mites, molds, animal fur, textile flooring, and smoke. A family history of atopic disease increases the probability of AR as the causative condition. Medications, including nonsteroidal anti-inflammatory drugs, aspirin,[6] antihypertensives, and topical nasal decongestants,[4] can precipitate or worsen symptoms. A review of systems should focus on identifying other comorbid conditions that suggest a diagnosis of AR, including asthma, conjunctivitis, sleep disorder, and otitis media. Often patients cannot distinguish symptoms caused by AR from the common cold, and the frequency and severity of these colds should be firmly established.

Although an accurate history is paramount in diagnosing AR, the physical examination is useful to help rule out other conditions or even concomitant pathology. Nasal mucosal swelling can lead to eustachian tube dysfunction, which manifests as a retracted immobile tympanic membrane with pneumatic otoscopy, although an ear examination is typically normal in patients with AR.[6]

Findings on anterior rhinoscopy may reveal an erythematous mucosa with swollen turbinates. The turbinates may appear to have the traditional bluish mother-of-pearl hue; however, this may be seen in non-AR as well.[9] Rhinoscopy is useful for determining the presence of a nasal polyp (NP) or deviated septum, both of which can cause airflow obstruction that patients may perceive as persistent congestion.

According to guidelines published by the American Academy of Otolaryngology - Head and Neck Surgery, allergy testing should be reserved for patients who (1) have a clinical diagnosis of AR but do not respond to empiric treatment or (2) require identification of the specific allergen to target therapy.[4] Allergy testing may be performed as a skin test or serum-specific IgE (SSIgE) level.

Clinical skin prick testing (SPT) has been in use for more than 100 years to aid in the diagnosis of atopic, IgE-mediated conditions and is considered the gold standard to which other diagnostic modalities are compared.

SPT has been validated as a safe and efficient means to diagnose allergy. With results available in 15 to 20 minutes, SPT allows for the evaluation of multiple allergens in a single session. SPT lancets and are designed to penetrate the stratum corneum, exposing the underlying epidermis to the allergen in question. Multiple site devices allow for testing of up to 10 different allergens in a single testing session. There are several variables that can affect the outcome of SPT. Controllable patient-dependent variables include anatomic testing site and distance between sites, whereas operator-dependent factors include technique affecting the angle and depth of penetration. Uncontrollable patient-related factors include age, race, or sun-damaged skin. Underlying comorbidities, such as an immunodeficiency, diabetes, or hypertension, can inhibit the immunologic response to SPT.[17]

Intradermal testing (IDT) involves the same principles as SPT; however, the allergen is introduced into the dermal skin layer using a standard hypodermic needle and syringe. IDT, although generally more sensitive and reproducible than SPT, is less well tolerated, takes longer to perform, and is associated with more false positive results. There is also a greater risk of systemic reactions with IDT as opposed to SPT. IDT is usually performed after a negative SPT.

The only absolute contraindications to SPT and IDT are recent anaphylaxis, pregnancy, certain medications that cannot be discontinued, and any form of extensive skin disease.

An alternative to in vivo skin testing is SSIgE levels. One advantage of SSIgE testing is the lack of interference from antihistamines or other medications. Disadvantages include the need to obtain blood, cost, and delays in test results.[18] A prospective study comparing SPT to SSIgE for 53 different inhalant allergens in patients with chronic rhinitis concluded that serum testing should be viewed as complementary and not equivalent to SPT.[19]

Once a diagnosis of AR is confirmed using a combination of history and physical and diagnostic testing, it is vital to properly stage the extent of disease because this helps guide treatment. AR was previously categorized as either seasonal (occurring during a particular time of year) or perennial (present throughout the entire year); however, this has been abandoned in favor of a classification similar to that used in asthma, which, as discussed previously, shares many features with AR. Symptoms are classified by duration as either intermittent (less than 6 weeks) or persistent and by symptom severity as either mild or moderate to severe. Mild symptoms do not interfere with sleep or daily activities whereas moderate to severe symptoms result in sleep derangements and in work/life impairment[6] (**Fig. 1**).

MANAGEMENT AND TREATMENT

There is an extensive armamentarium available to treat the symptoms of AR. Unfortunately, as a type 1 hypersensitivity-mediated process, there is no known cure. A majority of symptoms can be managed by a primary care provider, but

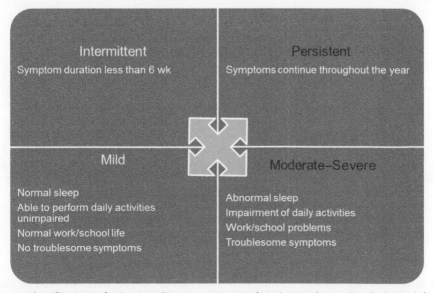

Fig. 1. Classification of AR according to symptom duration and severity. (*Adapted from* Small P, Kim H. Allergic rhinitis. Allergy Asthma Clin Immunol 2011;7(Suppl 1):S3.)

clinicians must remain vigilant for unusual presentations and red flag symptoms, prompting referral to an appropriate specialist.[20]

An overview of the stepwise treatment of AR is available in **Fig. 2**.[6] In general, management involves allergen avoidance, oral antihistamines, intranasal corticosteroids, leukotriene receptor antagonists, and, lastly, allergen immunotherapy with intranasal corticosteroids as the mainstay of treatment.

Exposure to relevant allergens and irritants, such as dust mites, molds, pollens, pets, and tobacco smoke, should be minimized. Effective strategies include allergen-impermeable bedding covers and keeping indoor relative humidity below 50% to inhibit mite growth. Pollen exposure can be minimized by limiting time spent outdoors and by keeping windows closed. Removing pets from the home can reduce symptoms within 4 to 6 months for patients who are allergic to animal dander.[6] Commercially available high-efficiency particulate air filters have been shown to reduce indoor levels of common asthma and allergy triggers.[21] Early studies suggested no improvement in symptoms, but multiple studies since 2000 have shown symptomatic benefit in both AR and asthma. Further research is needed to clearly define the effect of air filtration on AR-related disease outcomes.[22]

Nasal irrigation with isotonic saline has been shown effective according to a 2012 systematic review. Nasal symptoms decreased by an average of 27.66% and medicine consumption decreased by an average of 2.99%. Both saline nasal spray and high-volume (200–400 mL) irrigation showed symptomatic benefit.[23]

Oral antihistamines have years of proved efficacy in the treatment of AR. First-generation antihistamines include diphenhydramine and chlorpheniramine and are commonly used, both over the counter and through prescriptions. These older agents are not selective for the H_1-receptor. They cross the blood-brain barrier and have effects on dopamine, serotonin, and acetylcholine receptors. As such they

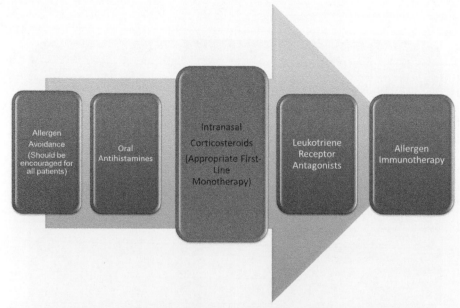

Fig. 2. A simplified, stepwise algorithm for the treatment of AR. Treatments can be used individually or in any combination. (*Adapted from* Small P, Kim H. Allergic rhinitis. Allergy Asthma Clin Immunol 2011;7(Suppl 1):S3.)

may cause a host of wanted side effects, including some that affect the central nervous system (CNS).

Newer-generation antihistamines include cetirizine, desloratadine, and fexofenadine. They are similar in efficacy to first-generation medications.[24] These agents have the benefit of an improved safety profile with reduced CNS effects as well as decreased incidence of cardiovascular side effects, such as prolonged QT. Placebo-controlled and head-to-head trials with these newer antihistamines have shown that they are statistically significantly better than placebo at reducing symptoms and have similar efficacy among themselves. Even these newer agents, however, can cause CNS effects at recommended doses. One study showed the combined incidence of drowsiness and fatigue was significantly greater in patients treated with cetirizine than in those treated with fexofenadine.[25] It has also been reported that up to 7% of the general population and 20% of the African American population may be slow metabolizers of desloratadine, increasing their risk of unwanted side effects. Among the newer-generation antihistamines, fexofenadine has the lowest risk of side effects, specifically sedation/impairment, even at a higher than recommended dose (Table 1).[24]

Intranasal corticosteroids are the single best therapy for AR and are recommended as first-line treatment of patients with mild to moderate persistent symptoms. They function by decreasing the inflammatory cellular response, thus inhibiting cytokine release, reducing mucus production, and decreasing leukotriene and prostaglandin response.[26] With an onset of action of 30 minutes, their effects can last for up to several hours. There are many available formulations, both prescription and over the counter, and no single one has been shown superior in either safety or efficacy. As a class, intranasal corticosteroids have the benefit of improving ocular symptoms related to allergic conjunctivitis.[26] Budesonide is the sole agent that carries an FDA pregnancy category B rating.[27] Despite their universally accepted efficacy, inhaled steroids do pose risks for patients. The most commonly reported adverse effects are headache, throat irritation, epistaxis, stinging, burning, and nasal dryness.[28] The rate of skeletal growth was unaffected in children treated using mometasone for

Table 1
Sedation associated with first-generation and second-generation antihistamines

Agent	Sedation/Impairment Effect	
	Recommended Dose	Above Recommended Dose
Diphenhydramine (first generation)	↑↑↑	↑↑↑
Clemastine (first generation)	↑↑↑	↑↑↑
Chlorpheniramine (first generation)	↑↑	↑↑
Cetirizine (second generation)	↑	↑↑
Desloratadine (second generation)	↔	↑
Fexofenadine (second generation)	↔	↔

Adapted from Spangler DL, Brunton S. Efficacy and central nervous system impairment of newer-generation prescription antihistamines in seasonal allergic rhinitis. South Med J 2006;99(6):594; with permission.

1 year in 1 randomized placebo-controlled trial.[29] A 2015 placebo-controlled study did reveal, however, a small yet statistically significant difference in growth velocity in children treated with 110 μg of intranasal triamcinolone (5.65 cm/y vs 6.09 cm/y). At 2-month follow-up, the growth velocity in the treatment group approached baseline growth rate, indicating a catch-up period on treatment cessation.[30]

Although FDA-approved treatment options for AR, the leukotriene receptor antagonists montelukast and zafirlukast offer only minimal improvement in nasal congestion. This was evidenced by a systematic review of 20 trials involving adults treated with montelukast.[31] Leukotriene receptor antagonists, although better than placebo, are inferior to intranasal corticosteroids and antihistamines and should be used as a second-line or third-line option.

Allergen immunotherapy is a proved long-term treatment option for AR. The risk of potentially life-threatening consequences of allergen immunotherapy is very low; nonetheless, it should only be prescribed by physicians who are adequately trained in allergy treatment and capable of managing anaphylaxis.[6] A patient's triggering allergens are administered either by subcutaneous immunotherapy (SCIT) or sublingual immunotherapy (SLIT). Doses are slowly increased every week for 6 to 8 months until immunologic tolerance is reached. Maintenance injections are then given every 3 to 4 weeks for 3 to 5 years at the maximum tolerated dose. Evidence supports use of immunotherapy for allergy to pollens and dust mites; mold and animal dander allergies are less responsive.[6] A 2009 Cochrane review of SCIT confirmed its efficacy and low side-effect profile; 0.56% of participants had events categorized as early systemic reaction grade 4, which refers to either respiratory failure with or without loss of consciousness or hypotension with or without loss of consciousness, with 1 of 4 of those events occurring after placebo administration. There were no fatalities reported.[32] SLIT is an alternative approach in providing allergen immunotherapy. It has been found better tolerated with lower dropout rates than SCIT due to its lower cost, ease of administration, and favorable side-effect profile. These factors, combined with its similar efficacy to SCIT, are making SLIT a more attractive option for patients and providers alike.[33]

Alternative therapeutic modalities include acupuncture, nasal air filters, intranasal carbon dioxide, intranasal cellulose, and homeopathy. Although many of these have shown positive results in small trials, they have not been adopted as recommended treatment strategies.[34]

CHRONIC RHINOSINUSITIS AND NASAL POLYPS

Chronic rhinosinusitis (CRS) with nasal polyposis or CRS without nasal polyposis is a clinical syndrome distinct from AR and is marked by nasal and paranasal inflammation with symptoms lasting longer than 3 months. Rhinosinusitis in adults is characterized by 2 or more symptoms, 1 of which should be either nasal blockage/congestion or nasal discharge, which can be anterior or posterior. Additional diagnostic symptoms include facial pain or pressure and reduction or loss of smell. This should be accompanied by endoscopic or CT changes of mucosal inflammation or polyposis.[35] Radiographic findings on CT include ostiomeatal complex or sinus mucosal changes. On endoscopy, NPs, mucopurulent discharge, edema, and mucosal obstruction may be seen.[36]

The most common category of CRS in Western countries is eosinophilic CRS, which encompasses several eosinophilic processes, including allergic fungal rhinosinusitis, eosinophilic mucin rhinosinusitis, eosinophilic fungal rhinosinusitis, and aspirin-exacerbated respiratory disease. Allergic fungal rhinosinusitis is an

IgE-mediated response to mold whereas there is no specific IgE response in eosinophilic mucin rhinosinusitis or eosinophilic fungal rhinosinusitis.[37]

NPs form as a result of chronic inflammation of the paranasal sinus mucosa. Typically benign, they usually develop bilaterally in adulthood. NPs found in children may be the presenting sign for cystic fibrosis whereas unilateral NPs should be evaluated for malignancy.[38] The prevalence of NP is approximately 4% with a 2:1 male-to-female ratio.[38] A majority of cases of nasal polyposis are idiopathic, but rare causes, such as Wegener granulomatosis and sarcoidosis, should be considered.[36]

Therapy for NP involves observation, medical therapies, and surgical interventions. The goals of medical treatment are to reduce nasal obstruction, improve sinus drainage, and restore olfaction and taste.[39] These can be accomplished with a combination of topical and/or systemic steroids, nasal saline irrigation, and long-term antibiotics. Surgery should be reserved for those patients who remain symptomatic despite maximum medical treatment.[36]

SUMMARY

As the most prevalent atopic condition affecting 10% to 20% of the population, AR deserves a thorough understanding of its manifestations, diagnosis, and treatment. Dismissed as trivial by many, AR is a source of profound distress for millions across the world, resulting in billions of dollars of lost productivity. Primary care providers should routinely screen for this condition because patients may view their symptoms as unavoidable and neglect to mention it.

A thorough history and physical examination are often sufficient to make the diagnosis. Further testing is available in the form of SPT and SSIgE measurements. These modalities are typically used when patients do not respond to initial treatment or if identification of a specific allergen is important to guide therapy.

Unfortunately, there is no cure for AR. Many treatment options are available, including oral medications, topical sprays, and SCIT or SLIT. Intranasal corticosteroids are the mainstay of treatment. Regardless of the therapeutic approach, allergen avoidance remains a vital component of any treatment plan.

CRS is a distinct clinical entity from AR but may also involve an atopic component depending on the subtype. The etiology of polyp formation in CRS remains unknown. Treatment CRS with or without NPs should focus on symptom relief, with surgery as an option for patients who have failed maximum medical therapy.

REFERENCES

1. Dykewicz MS, Hamilos DL. Rhinitis and sinusitis. J Allergy Clin Immunol 2010; 125:S103–15.
2. Stewart M, Ferguson BJ, Fromer L. Epidemiology and burden of nasal congestion. Int J Gen Med 2010;3:37–45.
3. Asher MI, Montefort S, Björkstén B, et al. Worldwide time trends in the prevalence of symptoms of asthma, allergic rhinoconjunctivitis, and eczema in childhood: ISAAXC Phase One and Three repeat multicountry cross-sectional surveys. Lancet 2006;368:733–43.
4. Seidman MD, Gurgel RK, Lin SY, et al. Clinical practice guideline: allergic rhinitis. Otolaryngol Head Neck Surg 2015;152(2):197–206.
5. Lamb CE, Ratner PH, Johnson CE, et al. Economic impact of workplace productivity losses due to allergic rhinitis compared with select medical conditions in the United States from an employer perspective. Curr Med Res Opin 2006;22:1203–10.
6. Small P, Kim H. Allergic rhinitis. Allergy Asthma Clin Immunol 2011;7(Suppl 1):S3.

7. Macy E. A rhinitis primer for family medicine. Perm J 2012;16(4):61–6.
8. Harkema JR, Carey SA, Wagner JG. The nose revisited: a brief review of the comparative structure, function, and toxicologic pathology of the nasal epithelium. Toxicol Pathol 2006;34(3):252–69.
9. Weber RW. Allergic rhinitis. Prim Care 2008;35(1):1–10.
10. Schatz M. A survey of the burden of allergic rhinitis in the USA. Allergy 2007; 62(Suppl 85):9–16.
11. Lakhani N, North M, Ellis AK. Clinical manifestations of allergic rhinitis. Journal Allergy Therapy 2012;S5:007.
12. Nathan RA. Management of patients with allergic rhinitis and asthma: literature review. South Med J 2009;102(9):935–41.
13. Ellegard EK. Clinical and pathogenetic characteristics of pregnancy rhinitis. Clin Rev Allergy Immunol 2004;26(3):149–59.
14. Scarupa MD, Kaliner MA. Nonallergic rhinitis, with a focus on vasomotor rhinitis: clinical importance, differential diagnosis, and effective treatment recommendations. World Allergy Organ J 2009;2(3):20–5.
15. Wheeler PW, Wheeler SF. Vasomotor rhinitis. Am Fam Physician 2005;72(6): 1057–62.
16. Min YG. The pathophysiology, diagnosis and treatment of allergic rhinitis. Allergy Asthma Immunol Res 2010;2(2):65–76.
17. Fatteh S, Rekkerth DJ, Hadley JA. Skin prick/puncture testing in North America: a call for standards and consistency. Allergy Asthma Clin Immunol 2014;10(1):44.
18. Sicherer SH, Wood RA. Allergy testing in childhood: using allergen-specific IgE tests. Pediatrics 2012;129(1):193–7.
19. Calabria CW, Dietrich J, Hagan L. Comparison of serum-specific IgE (ImmunoCAP) and skin-prick test results for 53 inhalant allergens in patients with chronic rhinitis. Allergy Asthma Proc 2009;30(4):386–96.
20. Angier E, Willington J, Scadding G, et al. Management of allergic and nonallergic rhinitis: a primary care summary of the BSACI guideline. Prim Care Respir J 2010;19(3):217–22.
21. Brown KW, Minegishi T, Allen JG, et al. Reducing patients' exposures to asthma and allergy triggers in their homes: an evaluation of effectiveness of grades of forced air ventilation filters. J Asthma 2014;51(6):585–94.
22. Sublett JL, Seltzer J, Burkhead R, et al. Air filters and air cleaners: rostrum by the American Academy of Allergy, Asthma & Immunology Indoor Allergen Committee. J Allergy Clin Immunol 2010;125(1):32–8.
23. Hermelingmeier KE, Weber RK, Hellmich M, et al. Nasal irrigation as an adjunctive treatment in allergic rhinitis: a systematic review and meta-analysis. Am J Rhinol Allergy 2012;26(5):e119–25.
24. Spangler DL, Brunton S. Efficacy and central nervous system impairment of newer-generation prescription antihistamines in seasonal allergic rhinitis. South Med J 2006;99(6):593–9.
25. Howarth PH, Stern MA, Roi L, et al. Double-blind, placebo-controlled study comparing the efficacy and safety of fexofenadine hydrochloride (120 mg and 180 mg once-daily) and cetirizine in seasonal allergic rhinitis. J Allergy Clin Immunol 1999;104:927–33.
26. Okano M. Mechanisms and clinical implications of glucocorticosteroids in the treatment of allergic rhinitis. Clin Exp Immunol 2009;158(2):164–73.
27. Sur DK, Scandale S. Treatment of Allergic Rhinitis. Am Fam Physician 2010; 81(12):1440–6.

28. Demoly P. Safety of intranasal corticosteroids in acute rhinosinusitis. Am J Otolaryngol 2008;29(6):403–13.
29. Schenkel EJ, Skoner DP, Bronsky EA, et al. Absence of growth retardation in children with perennial allergic rhinitis after one year of treatment with mometasone furoate aqueous nasal spray. Pediatrics 2000;105(2):E22.
30. Skoner DP, Berger WE, Gawchik SM, et al. Intranasal triamcinolone and growth velocity. Pediatrics 2015;135:e348.
31. Grainger J, Drake-Lee A. Montelukast in allergic rhinitis: a systematic review and meta-analysis. Clin Otolaryngol 2006;31(5):360–7.
32. Calderon MA, Alves B, Jacobson M, et al. Allergen injection immunotherapy for seasonal allergic rhinitis. Cochrane Database Syst Rev 2007;(1):CD001936.
33. Aboshady OA, Elghanam KM. Sublingual immunotherapy in allergic rhinitis: efficacy, safety, adherence and guidelines. Clin Exp Otorhinolaryngol 2014;7(4):241–9.
34. Solelhac G, Charpin D. Management of allergic rhinitis. F1000prime Rep 2014;6:94.
35. Fokkens WJ, Lund VJ, Mullol J, et al. EPOS 2012: European position paper on rhinosinusitis and nasal polyps 2012. A summary for otorhinolaryngologists. Rhinology 2012;50:1–12.
36. Piromchai P, Kasemsiri P, Laohasiriwong S, et al. Chronic rhinosinusitis and emerging treatment options. Int J Gen Med 2013;6:453–64.
37. Chaaban MR, Walsh EM, Woodworth BA. Epidemiology and differential diagnosis of nasal polyps. Am J Rhinol Allergy 2013;27(6):473–8.
38. Stevens WW, Schleimer RP, Chandra RK. Biology of nasal polyposis. J Allergy Clin Immunol 2014;133(5):1503, 1503.e1-4.
39. Newton JR, Ah-See KW. A review of nasal polyposis. Ther Clin Risk Manag 2008; 4(2):507–12.

Anaphylaxis

Lorenzo Hernandez, MD, MS[a], Sarah Papalia, MD[a],
George G.A. Pujalte, MD[b],*

KEYWORDS

- Anaphylaxis • Shock • IgE • Hypersensitivity • Allergen • Bronchospasm
- Angioedema • Epinephrine

KEY POINTS

- Anaphylaxis is an immunoglobulin E–mediated hypersensitivity reaction that can potentially lead to death.
- An increasing incidence is presumed to be related to food processing practices.
- Diagnostic tests lack specificity; thus, it is imperative that a clinical diagnosis be made and treatment initiated as soon as possible.
- The definition requires the involvement of multiple organ systems, which include the respiratory, gastrointestinal, cardiovascular, and central nervous systems.
- The best treatment plan is one of prevention and efforts should be focused on recognition of triggers and implementing personalized action plans.

INTRODUCTION

Anaphylaxis is an acute, shocklike, and potentially fatal state. It occurs owing to the release of bioactive factors from mast cells and basophils and is a response to antigenic sensitivity. Portier and Richet coined the term in 1903[1] after attempts to vaccinate dogs using jelly fish toxin resulted in fatal sensitivity reactions rather than protective properties. The term reflects the antiprophylactic effect, and the concept was found deserving of the Nobel Prize in 1913. Although presentation of the condition varies, dermatologic manifestations are the initial symptom in a majority of adult patients. Children are more likely to present with respiratory symptoms followed by cutaneous symptoms. Other systems commonly affected by anaphylaxis include the cardiovascular, gastrointestinal, and neurologic systems. Diagnostic tests, including serum tryptase and serum-specific immunoglobulin (Ig)E, lack specificity; thus, it is imperative that a clinical diagnosis be made efficiently. Treatment mainstays include epinephrine, antihistamines, fluid resuscitation, and airway management, which must be initiated immediately to minimize morbidity and mortality. Prevention efforts focus on awareness and recognition of triggers and educating patients about the

[a] Department of Family Medicine, Mayo Clinic, 4500 San Pablo Rd, Jacksonville, FL 32224, USA;
[b] Department of Family Medicine, Mayo Clinic College of Medicine, Mayo Clinic, 4500 San Pablo Rd, Jacksonville, FL 32224, USA
* Corresponding author.
E-mail address: Pujalte.George@mayo.edu

Prim Care Clin Office Pract 43 (2016) 477–485
http://dx.doi.org/10.1016/j.pop.2016.04.002
0095-4543/16/$ – see front matter © 2016 Elsevier Inc. All rights reserved.
primarycare.theclinics.com

implementation of personalized action plans. The incidence of anaphylaxis has significantly increased over the past 10 years, particularly in the pediatric population, a change that is the focus of numerous ongoing studies.

PATHOPHYSIOLOGY OVERVIEW

Like more benign localized atopy such as food allergy and asthma, systemic anaphylactic responses are classified as IgE-mediated hypersensitivity reactions. This type of reaction begins when IgE bound to B-cells makes contact with an antigen, leading to the production of large amounts of antigen-specific IgE, which are clustered on the surface of mast cells and basophils. Subsequent exposure to the antigen leads to the release of immune-modulating factors, such as leukotrienes and histamine, from the primed immune cells.[2] Downstream effects include systemic smooth muscle contraction, vasodilation, and bronchiole constriction, which give way to hypotensive shock and asphyxiation, the main causes of morbidity and mortality.[3] Sympathetic activation with epinephrine directly counteracts these effects by causing smooth muscle relaxation, vasoconstriction, increasing cardiac output, and blocking further degranulation on a biomolecular level by increasing cyclic adenosine monophosphate.[2]

RISK FACTORS

Atopy is the genetic propensity for the development of immediate hypersensitivity reactions and is the single most important risk factor for anaphylaxis. It is believed to be multigenic and has known associations with several genes, including those for cytokines and the IgE receptor, and suspected associations with unidentified genes.[4] Numerous other individual factors have been shown to influence the severity of the reaction (**Table 1**). Medications such as beta-blockers, angiotensin-converting enzyme inhibitors, diuretics, and antihypertensives in aggregate increase the risk for severe reactions owing to compounded hypotension and bronchospasm.

INCIDENCE AND CAUSATIVE AGENTS

Although anaphylaxis is recognized as a relatively common reaction and potentially lethal condition, data are limited regarding the prevalence and characteristics in the

Table 1	
Factors increasing risk for anaphylaxis severity and fatality	
Risk Factor	**Cause of Severity and Fatality**
Age	Infants: underdiagnoses, no action plan
	Pregnancy: antibiotic therapy
Medications	Affect recognition of symptoms: sedatives, hypnotics, recreational drugs
Comorbidities	Asthma, pulmonary disease
	Mastocytosis
	Thyroid disease: associated with idiopathic form
Other	Exercise, acute infection, menses, hyperhistaminemia, reduced level of ACE or PAF AH activity

Abbreviations: ACE, angiotensin-converting enzyme; AH, acetylhydrolase; PAF, platelet-activating factor.

Data from Lang DM. Do beta-blockers really enhance the risk of anaphylaxis during immunotherapy? Curr Allergy Asthma Rep 2008;8(1):37–44; and Bonadonna P, Perbellini O, Passalacqua G, et al. Clonal mast cell disorders in patients with systemic reactions to hymenoptera stings and increased serum tryptase levels. J Allergy Clin Immunol 2009;123(3):680–6.

general population. Some clinicians reserve the term for the full-blown syndrome, whereas others use it to describe milder cases with any systemic involvement.

Regardless of how the condition is defined, it is widely accepted that, in Western countries, food-induced anaphylaxis, in particular, has increased at least 2-fold in prevalence over the past 20 years. Although partially owing to increased awareness and recognition, genetic studies have shown the increase to be attributable partly to new allergens that are the result of modern food processing methods.[5] This is 1 area of focus for current and future studies.

Wood and colleagues[3] first reported results of 2 nationwide surveys, which provided the first estimate of prevalence using large, stringently defined, unbiased results. It was concluded that lifetime prevalence is at least 1.6%. This is likely a grossly underestimated value owing to misdiagnosis and underreporting, particularly when symptoms are mild or transient.[6]

The most common triggers are outlined below and vary based on population source (**Table 2**). Severe food allergy is more common in children than in adults.[7] However, the frequency in adults may be increasing, because this and other forms of atopy often persist into adulthood. Episodes of anaphylaxis occur more frequently from July through September, a difference that is attributable to insect stings.[5] Reactions to insects and other venomous plants and animals are more prevalent in tropical areas because of the greater biodiversity in these areas. Exposure, and therefore reactions, to medications are more common in industrialized areas. Idiopathic anaphylaxis is described as a recurrent reaction, for which no consistent trigger can be determined, despite an exhaustive search.[8] It is most common in female patients with a known history of atopy.[8] Two-thirds of patients have 5 or fewer episodes per year, whereas one-third have more than 5 episodes per year.

CLINICAL PRESENTATION

Clinical presentation and assessment are important in the diagnosis of anaphylaxis. Characteristic symptoms and signs of anaphylaxis can involve several different organ systems, and they differ from one patient to another.[9] These organ systems include the respiratory, gastrointestinal, cardiovascular, and central nervous systems.

Skin

Skin manifestations include flushing, itching, urticaria (hives), angioedema, morbilliform rash, pilor erection, periorbital itching, erythema and edema, conjunctival erythema, tearing, itching of the lips, tongue, palate, and external auditory canals, swelling of the lips, tongue and uvula, and itching of the genitalia, palms, and/or soles.

Table 2	
Documented triggers of severe anaphylaxis in adult and pediatric populations	
Adult	**Pediatric**
Foods (32%): Seafood, nuts, milk, egg, sesame	Foods (85%): Seafood, nuts, milk
Insect venom (19%): Bee, wasp, hornet, ant	Insect venom (4%): Bee, wasp, hornet, ant
Medications (35%): Beta lactam antibiotics, nonsteroidal antiinflammatory drugs, insulin, antitoxins, chemotherapy	Unknown (11%)
Unknown (14%)	

Data from Lieberman P. Anaphylaxis. 7th edition. St Louis: Mosby, Inc.; 2009; and Wood RA, Camargo Jr CA, Lieberman P, et al. Anaphylaxis in America: the prevalence and characteristics of anaphylaxis in the United States. J Allergy Clin Immunol 2014;133(2):461–7.

Respiratory

Respiratory symptoms include nasal itching, congestion, rhinorrhea, sneezing, throat itching and tightness, dysphonia, hoarseness, stridor, dry staccato cough, cyanosis, and respiratory arrest.

Lower Airways

Lower airway symptoms include increased respiratory rate, shortness of breath, chest tightness, deep cough, wheezing/bronchospasm, and decreased peak expiratory flow.

Gastrointestinal

Gastrointestinal symptoms include abdominal pain, nausea, vomiting (stringy mucus), diarrhea, and dysphagia.

Cardiovascular

Cardiovascular manifestations include chest pain, tachycardia, bradycardia (less common), other arrhythmias, palpitations, hypotension, feeling faint, urinary or fecal incontinence, shock, and cardiac arrest.

Central Nervous System

Central nervous system symptoms include an aura of impending doom, uneasiness (in infants and children, sudden behavioral change, eg, irritability, cessation of play, clinging to parent; throbbing headache (before epinephrine), altered mental status, dizziness, confusion, and tunnel vision.

Other

Other symptoms may include a metallic taste in the mouth and cramps and bleeding owing to uterine contractions in females.

Skin signs are present in 80% to 90% of all patients and, when they are absent, anaphylaxis is more difficult to recognize. Respiratory tract involvement is seen in up to 70% of patients, while the gastrointestinal tract and cardiovascular system are present in up to 45%. Central nervous system involvement is seen in up to 15% of patients. At the beginning of an episode, it can be difficult to predict the rate of progression or the ultimate severity. Fatality can occur within minutes.[9–12]

The presentation of symptoms may also vary by age. In infancy, anaphylaxis can be difficult to recognize. Some of the signs associated with anaphylaxis are daily occurrences in babies, such as flushing and dysphonia after crying, spitting up after feeding, and incontinence.[11] Teens are vulnerable to anaphylaxis recurrences owing to risk-taking behaviors, such as failure to avoid their trigger(s) and failure to carry self-injectable epinephrine.[11]

Middle-aged and elderly patients are at increased risk for severe or fatal anaphylaxis because of known or subclinical cardiovascular diseases and the medications used to treat those conditions.[13] In the healthy human heart, mast cells are present around the coronary arteries and the intramural vessels, between the myocardial fibers, and in the arterial intima.[14] In patients with ischemic heart disease, the number and density of cardiac mast cells are increased in these areas. In addition, mast cells are present in the atherosclerotic plaques. During anaphylaxis, histamine, leukotrienes, platelet-activating factor and other mediators released from cardiac mast cells contribute to vasoconstriction and coronary artery spasm.[14]

DIFFERENTIAL DIAGNOSIS

In anaphylaxis, some of the most common diagnostic dilemmas involve acute asthma, syncope, and anxiety/panic attacks.[7,11,12,15] A severe asthma episode can cause diagnostic confusion because wheezing, coughing, and shortness of breath can occur in both asthma and anaphylaxis; however, itching, urticaria, angioedema, abdominal pain, and hypotension are unlikely in acute asthma. Similarly, an anxiety or panic attack can cause a diagnosis of confusion because a sense of impending doom, breathlessness, flushing, tachycardia, and gastrointestinal symptoms; these manifestations can occur in both anxiety or panic attacks and in anaphylaxis, but urticaria, angioedema, wheezing, and hypotension are unlikely during an anxiety or panic attack. Syncope (fainting) can cause diagnostic confusion because hypotension can occur; however, syncope is relieved by recumbency and is usually associated with pallor and sweating; urticaria, flushing, and respiratory symptoms, as well as gastrointestinal symptoms, are usually absent.[7,10,11]

Postprandial syndromes (scombroidosis, pollen–food allergy, monosodium glutamate, sulfites, food poisoning), excess endogenous histamine syndromes (myocytosis/clonal mast cell disorders, basophilic leukemia), flush syndromes (perimenopause, carcinoid, autonomic epilepsy, medullary carcinoma of the thyroid), nonorganic diseases (vocal cord dysfunction, hyperventilation, psychosomatic episode), and other diseases (nonallergic angioedema, hereditary angioedema, angiotensin-converting enzyme inhibitor–associated angioedema, systemic capillary leak syndrome, red man syndrome owing to vancomycin, pheochromocytoma) should also be considered in the differential diagnosis.[7,10–12,15]

DIAGNOSIS

A clinical diagnosis of anaphylaxis is based on consideration of the patient's presenting symptoms and signs and on ruling out other sudden-onset multisystem diseases.[16] Anaphylaxis is highly likely when any one of the following 3 criteria are fulfilled.[9,11]

- Acute onset of an illness (multiple to several hours) with involvement of the skin, mucosal tissue, or both (eg, generalized urticaria, itching or flushing, swollen lips-tongue-uvula) AND at least one of the following:
  - Respiratory compromise (eg, dyspnea, wheeze–bronchospasm, stridor, reduced peak expiratory flow, hypoxemia) or
  - Reduced blood pressure or associated symptoms of end-organ dysfunction (eg, hypotonia [collapse], syncope, incontinence).[9,11]
- Two or more of the following that occur rapidly after exposure to a likely allergen for that patient (minutes to several hours):
  - Involvement of the skin mucosal tissue (eg, generalized urticaria, itch–flush, swollen lips–tongue–uvula)
  - Respiratory compromise (eg, dyspnea, wheeze–bronchospasm, stridor, reduced peak expiratory flow, hypoxemia)
  - Reduced blood pressure or associated symptoms of end-organ dysfunction (eg, hypotonia [collapse], syncope, incontinence)
  - Persistent gastrointestinal symptoms (eg, crampy abdominal pain, vomiting)[9,11]
- Reduced blood pressure after exposure to known allergen for that patient (minutes to several hours):
  - Infants and children: low systolic blood pressure (age-specific), or a decrease in systolic blood pressure of greater than 30%

o Adults: systolic blood pressure of less than 90 mm Hg or greater than 30% decrease from patient's baseline.[9,11]

Laboratory tests also have an important role in the diagnosis of anaphylaxis. Blood samples for measurement of tryptase levels are optimally obtained 15 minutes to 3 hours after symptom onset. Blood samples for measurement of histamine levels are optimally obtained 15 to 60 minutes after symptom onset. These tests are not universally available, not performed on an emergent basis, and not specific for anaphylaxis.[10,11,16,17]

Increased serum tryptase levels often support a clinical diagnosis of anaphylaxis from insect stings or injected medications and in patients who are hypotensive; however, levels are often within normal limits in patients with anaphylaxis triggered by food an in those who are normotensive.[11,18] Serial measurements of tryptase levels during an anaphylactic episode and measurement of a baseline level after recovery are reported to be more useful than measurement at only 1 point in time.[10,17] Normal levels of either tryptase or histamine do not rule out the clinical diagnosis of anaphylaxis.[17,18] It has been found that transient increases in platelet-activating factor correlate better with anaphylaxis severity than tryptase or histamine concentrations do; however, platelet-activating factor concentrations return to baseline within 15 to 20 minutes.[16,19]

MANAGEMENT AND TREATMENT

Anaphylaxis is a medical emergency that requires a systemic approach in both assessment and management. In the preliminary stages, there should be a posted, written emergency protocol for recognition or treatment of anaphylaxis; this protocol should be rehearsed regularly. All triggers should be removed if possible. For example, an intravenous diagnostic or therapeutic agent that seems to be triggering symptoms should be discontinued. There should also be an assessment of the patient's circulation, airways, breathing, mental status, skin, and body weight (mass).

In addition to and in conjunction with these preliminary actions, any available assistance should be obtained from other medical units (eg, resuscitation team in hospital or other health care setting, or emergency medical services in community setting). The patient should also be given epinephrine (adrenaline) intramuscularly in the middle anterolateral aspect of the thigh, 0.01 mg/kg of a 1:1000 (1 mg/mL) solution, to a maximum of 0.5 mg (adult) or 0.3 mg (child). The time of the dose should be recorded and a repeat injection may be given in 5 to 15 minutes, if needed; most patients respond to 1 or 2 doses. The patient should be placed on the back or in a position of comfort if there is respiratory distress and/or vomiting. The lower extremities should be elevated, because fatality can occur within seconds if a patient stands or sits suddenly.[12]

When indicated at any time during the episode, high-flow supplemental oxygen (6–8 L/min) should be given by facemask or oropharyngeal airway. In addition, intravenous access should be established using needles or catheters with wide-bore cannulae (14–16 gauge for adults). One to 2 liters of 0.9% (isotonic) saline should be given rapidly (eg, 5–10 mL/kg in the first 5–10 minutes to an adult, or 10 mL/kg to a child). Cardiopulmonary resuscitation with continuous chest compressions should be initiated. At frequent and regular intervals, a patient's blood pressure, cardiac rate and function, respiratory status and oxygenation should be monitored, electrocardiograms should be ordered, and continuous noninvasive monitoring should be started, if possible.[10–12,15,16]

Anaphylaxis guidelines published to date in indexed, peer-reviewed journals differ in their recommendations for administration of second-line medications such as antihistamines, beta-2 adrenergic agonists, and glucocorticoids. The evidence base for the use of these medications in the initial management of anaphylaxis, including doses and dose regimens, is extrapolated primarily from their use in treatment of other diseases such as urticaria (antihistamines) or acute asthma (beta-2 adrenergic agonists and glucocorticoids). There is some concern that injecting 1 or more second-line medication potentially delays prompt injection of epinephrine, the first-line treatment.[9–12,15,20,21]

Few patients do not respond to timely, basic initial anaphylaxis treatment with epinephrine by intramuscular injection(s), positioning on the back with lower extremities elevated, supplemental oxygen, intravenous fluid resuscitation, and second-line medications. If possible, such patients should be transferred promptly to the care of a specialist team in emergency medicine, critical care medicine, or anesthesiology.[12] These patients may require intubation, intravenous vasopressors, or new interventions such as methylene blue, which has been successful, especially in patients with distributive shock and profound vasodilation.[22,23]

After apparent resolution of symptoms, duration of monitoring in a medically supervised setting should be individualized. For example, patients with moderated respiratory or cardiovascular compromise should be monitored for at least 4 hours and, if indicated, for 8 to 10 hours or longer; patients with severe or partnered anaphylaxis might require monitoring and interventions for days. In reality, local conditions, including the availability of trained and experienced staff and emergency department beds or hospital beds, often determine the duration of monitoring that is possible.[9,24–26]

PREVENTION

Medications can be used to prevent additional episodes. This includes providing self-injectable epinephrine/adrenaline from an autoinjector. One alternative to this is to provide self-injectable epinephrine from an ampule/syringe or prefilled syringe; this, however, is not a preferred formulation. Other aspects of discharge management include an anaphylaxis emergency action plan (personalized, written); medical identification (eg, bracelet, wallet card); medical record electronic flag or chart sticker; and an emphasis on the importance of follow-up investigations, preferably by an allergy or immunology specialist.

An assessment of sensitization to allergens is another key preventative measure. Before discharge from the emergency department, the measurement of allergen-specific levels of IgE in serum should be considered; this will allow for the assessment of sensitization to relevant allergens ascertained from the history of the anaphylactic episode. At least 3 to 4 weeks after the episode, allergen sensitization should be confirmed using skin tests to relevant allergens; if these tests are negative in a patient with a convincing history of anaphylaxis, repeating them weeks or months later should be considered. A challenge/provocation test (eg, with food or medication) might also be needed to assess the risk for future anaphylaxis episodes. Tests should be conducted only in well-equipped health care settings staffed by trained experienced professionals.

Long-term risk reduction measures include avoidance and/or immune modulation. In cases of food-triggered anaphylaxis, patients should be advised to practice strict avoidance of relevant food(s). Patients whose anaphylaxis is triggered by stinging insect venom should avoid those insects and undergo subcutaneous venom immunotherapies, which protects 80% to 90% of adults and 98% of children against anaphylaxis from future stings.[12] In cases of medication-triggered anaphylaxis, there should be an avoidance of relevant medications and use of safe substitutes; if indicated, desensitization (using a published protocol) should be conducted in a health care setting as described. When patients present with idiopathic anaphylaxis (anaphylaxis of unknown etiology), there should be a search for hidden or novel triggers; baseline tryptase concentrations should be measured to help identify mast cell activation disorders, and glucocorticoid and H1-antihistamine prophylaxis for 2 to 3 months should be considered. Finally, there should be optimal management of asthma and other concomitant diseases.[7–10,12,15,27–38]

REFERENCES

1. Lieberman P. Anaphylaxis. 7th edition. St Louis (MO): Mosby, Inc.; 2009.
2. McCance KL, Huether SE. Pathophysiology: the biologic basis for disease in adults and children. 6th edition. Toronto (United Kingdom): Mosby; 2010.
3. Wood RA, Camargo CA Jr, Lieberman P, et al. Anaphylaxis in America: the prevalence and characteristics of anaphylaxis in the United States. J Allergy Clin Immunol 2014;133(2):461–7.
4. Kindt TJ, Goldsby RA, Osborne BA, et al. Kuby Immunology. Macmillan; 2007.
5. Koplin JJ, Mills EN, Allen KJ. Epidemiology of food allergy and food-induced anaphylaxis: is there really a Western world epidemic? Curr Opin Allergy Clin Immunol 2015;15(5):409–16.
6. Simons FE, Sampson HA. Anaphylaxis epidemic: fact or fiction? J Allergy Clin Immunol 2008;122(6):1166–8.
7. Simons FE. Anaphylaxis. J Allergy Clin Immunol 2010;125(2 Suppl 2):S161–81.
8. Greenberger PA, Lieberman P. Idiopathic anaphylaxis. J Allergy Clin Immunol Pract 2014;2(3):243–50 [quiz: 251].
9. Sampson HA, Munoz-Furlong A, Campbell RL, et al. Second symposium on the definition and management of anaphylaxis: summary report–second national institute of allergy and infectious disease/food allergy and anaphylaxis network symposium. J Allergy Clin Immunol 2006;117(2):391–7.
10. Lieberman P, Nicklas RA, Oppenheimer J, et al. The diagnosis and management of anaphylaxis practice parameter: 2010 update. J Allergy Clin Immunol 2010; 126(3):477–80.e1–42.
11. Simons FE, Ardusso LR, Bilo MB, et al. World Allergy Organization guidelines for the assessment and management of anaphylaxis. World Allergy Organ J 2011; 4(2):13–37.
12. Brown SG, Mullins RJ, Gold MS. Anaphylaxis: diagnosis and management. Med J Aust 2006;185(5):283–9.
13. Lieberman P, Simons FE. Anaphylaxis and cardiovascular disease: therapeutic dilemmas. Clin Exp Allergy 2015;45(8):1288–95.
14. Triggiani M, Patella V, Staiano RI, et al. Allergy and the cardiovascular system. Clin Exp Immunol 2008;153(Suppl 1):7–11.
15. Soar J, Pumphrey R, Cant A, et al. Emergency treatment of anaphylactic reactions–guidelines for healthcare providers. Resuscitation 2008;77(2):157–69.
16. Simons FE, Ardusso LR, Dimov V, et al. World Allergy Organization anaphylaxis guidelines: 2013 update of the evidence base. Int Arch Allergy Immunol 2013; 162(3):193–204.
17. Komarow HD, Hu Z, Brittain E, et al. Serum tryptase levels in atopic and nonatopic children. J Allergy Clin Immunol 2009;124(4):845–8.
18. Simons FE, Frew AJ, Ansotegui IJ, et al. Practical allergy (PRACTALL) report: risk assessment in anaphylaxis. Allergy 2008;63(1):35–7.

19. Vadas P, Perelman B, Liss G. Platelet-activating factor, histamine, and tryptase levels in human anaphylaxis. J Allergy Clin Immunol 2013;131(1):144-9.
20. Sheikh A, Ten Broek V, Brown SG, et al. H1-antihistamines for the treatment of anaphylaxis: Cochrane systematic review. Allergy 2007;62(8):830-7.
21. Choo KJ, Simons FE, Sheikh A. Glucocorticoids for the treatment of anaphylaxis. Evid Based Child Health 2013;8(4):1276-94.
22. Jang DH, Nelson LS, Hoffman RS. Methylene blue for distributive shock: a potential new use of an old antidote. J Med Toxicol 2013;9(3):242-9.
23. Bauer CS, Vadas P, Kelly KJ. Methylene blue for the treatment of refractory anaphylaxis without hypotension. Am J Emerg Med 2013;31(1):264.e3-e5.
24. Oswalt ML, Kemp SF. Anaphylaxis: office management and prevention. Immunol Allergy Clin North Am 2007;27(2):177-91, vi.
25. Kemp SF, Lockey RF, Simons FE, et al. Epinephrine: the drug of choice for anaphylaxis. A statement of the World Allergy Organization. Allergy 2008;63(8):1061-70.
26. Simons FE, World Allergy O. World Allergy Organization survey on global availability of essentials for the assessment and management of anaphylaxis by allergy-immunology specialists in health care settings. Ann Allergy Asthma Immunol 2010;104(5):405-12.
27. Lieberman P, Decker W, Camargo CA Jr, et al. SAFE: a multidisciplinary approach to anaphylaxis education in the emergency department. Ann Allergy Asthma Immunol 2007;98(6):519-23.
28. Muraro A, Roberts G, Clark A, et al. The management of anaphylaxis in childhood: position paper of the European academy of allergology and clinical immunology. Allergy 2007;62(8):857-71.
29. Nurmatov U, Worth A, Sheikh A. Anaphylaxis management plans for the acute and long-term management of anaphylaxis: a systematic review. J Allergy Clin Immunol 2008;122(2):353-61.e1-3.
30. Bilo MB, Bonifazi F. The natural history and epidemiology of insect venom allergy: clinical implications. Clin Exp Allergy 2009;39(10):1467-76.
31. Loibl M, Schwarz S, Ring J, et al. Definition of an exercise intensity threshold in a challenge test to diagnose food-dependent exercise-induced anaphylaxis. Allergy 2009;64(10):1560-1.
32. Mirakian R, Ewan PW, Durham SR, et al. BSACI guidelines for the management of drug allergy. Clin Exp Allergy 2009;39(1):43-61.
33. Nowak-Wegrzyn A, Assa'ad AH, Bahna SL, et al. Work group report: oral food challenge testing. J Allergy Clin Immunol 2009;123(Suppl 6):S365-83.
34. Joint Task Force on Practice Parameters, American Academy of Allergy, Asthma and Immunology, et al. Drug allergy: an updated practice parameter. Ann Allergy Asthma Immunol 2010;105(4):259-73.
35. Muller UR. Insect venoms. Chem Immunol Allergy 2010;95:141-56.
36. Simons KJ, Simons FE. Epinephrine and its use in anaphylaxis: current issues. Curr Opin Allergy Clin Immunol 2010;10(4):354-61.
37. Golden DB, Moffitt J, Nicklas RA, et al. Stinging insect hypersensitivity: a practice parameter update 2011. J Allergy Clin Immunol 2011;127(4):852-4.e1-23.
38. Sampson HA, Aceves S, Bock SA, et al. Food allergy: a practice parameter update-2014. J Allergy Clin Immunol 2014;134(5):1016-25.e43.

Allergen Immunotherapy

Efren Rael, MD

KEYWORDS

- Allergy immunotherapy • Standard subcutaneous immunotherapy (SCIT)
- Food immunotherapy • Venom immunotherapy (VIT) • Aeroallergen

KEY POINTS

- Allergies affect a large proportion of the population.
- Allergies can adversely affect productivity, sleep, and quality of life and can lead to life-threatening reactions.
- Allergies can spread to affect multiple organ systems.
- Allergen immunotherapy (AIT) is the only therapy that can change the natural history of allergic disease.

INTRODUCTION

Allergies in general affect a large percentage of the global population. There is wide variability in methods reporting allergic rhinitis prevalence, ranging from 8.4% of children and 7.7% of adults affected in the United States[1,2] to up to 40% affected worldwide.[3] Asthma affects 18.7 million American adults or 8% of the adult population and 6.8 million children or 9.3% of the pediatric population[?] and affects 20% of the European population.[4] Skin allergy affects 12.5% of the United States population under 18 years of age[5] and 15% of the European population.[4]

Food allergy prevalence and food-triggered anaphylaxis have increased over the past 2 decades as reported in a study comparing 2011 to 2012 with 2004 to 2005, in age groups 0 to 4 years and 5 to 14 years,[6] with additional studies supporting these findings.[7–9] The Centers for Disease Control/National Center for Health Statistics report 5% prevalence of food allergy in individuals under 18 years of age.[5] Indirect and direct costs associated with food allergy in children and adolescents are large. Management of pediatric food allergy increased total household costs in a European cohort by €3961 in children and €4792 in adolescents.[10]

Life-threatening stinging insect allergy affects 0.4% to 0.8% of children and 3% of adults.[11] Stinging insect allergy accounts for greater than 10% of anaphylaxis cases.[12]

AIT is the only therapy that can change the underlying natural history of the allergic conditions discussed previously and has been around for more than 100 years in various forms to treat allergy.[13,14] Pharmacologic therapies and allergen avoidance

Sean N. Parker Center for Allergy and Asthma Research, Stanford University, Box 18885, Stanford, CA 94309, USA
E-mail address: efrenrael@gmail.com

Prim Care Clin Office Pract 43 (2016) 487–494
http://dx.doi.org/10.1016/j.pop.2016.04.004
primarycare.theclinics.com
0095-4543/16/$ – see front matter © 2016 Elsevier Inc. All rights reserved.

measures can temporarily decrease symptoms; however, once discontinuation of these measures occurs, the immune system often reverts back to the allergic state.

DIAGNOSIS

- History
- Allergy testing
- Outside of food allergy, allergen challenge is usually not performed to confirm the diagnosis.
- Food challenge is confirmatory for the diagnosis of food allergy but should be done by a specialist with hospital support in the event anaphylaxis management is required.

The history is imperative to the diagnosis of allergic disease. Allergy history often consists of a sensitization phase, whereby the immune system establishes recognition of an allergen, followed in time by an effector phase, by which the immune system can respond to an allergen challenge and memory is established.[15]

Allergies often lead to a history of itch, mucus production, and swelling on allergen challenge. Allergies commonly affect the exposure site in a sensitized individual. For example, inhaled allergens can affect the upper and/or lower respiratory systems on allergen challenge[16] and can elicit symptoms of sneezing, itchy nose, rhinorrhea, and nasal congestion in the upper respiratory tract. In an asthmatic, symptoms can include cough, wheeze, shortness of breath, and chest tightness on allergen challenge.

Beyond allergic reaction development at the interface exposure site (such as the skin, eyes, and respiratory mucosa), once memory is established, if an allergen is able to get past a body barrier interface, circulating IgE allergic antibodies in the bloodstream can be a catalyst for more advanced systemic reactions. Allergens can bypass the natural barrier interface through capillaries under the tongue, absorption from the gastrointestinal tract, or injection from a stinging insect (such as a honey bee, wasp, hornet, yellow jacket, or fire ant). Food allergens, stinging insect venom allergens, and, less commonly asthma, can lead to life-threatening allergic reactions.

Once the history is suggestive, testing can help identify the allergen to which an individual is sensitized. Testing can be accomplished via a skin test or a blood test. For inhaled allergens and venom allergy diagnosis, allergen challenge is not usually required. In the setting of food allergy, however, some foods have components that are cross-reactive with environmental pollens and can elicit minor symptoms, such as mouth itch, thereby making it difficult to determine if there is true food allergy or a bystander effect from shared pollen allergen epitopes. As a result, food allergy skin and blood tests are not reliably accurate to confirm a diagnosis of food allergy, and indiscriminant food allergy testing without an allergy history can lead to unnecessary food avoidance, psychological angst for families, and, in severe cases, nutritional deficiencies. Hence, a food challenge to the suspected food associated with allergy symptoms is the gold standard for diagnosing food allergy. Food challenges should be conducted in a hospital setting by an expert in the field, in the event that emergent management with autoinjectable epinephrine and fluid resuscitation is required.

TYPES OF IMMUNOTHERAPY

- Aeroallergen, stinging insect venom, food
- Food immunotherapy is evolving.
- Standard and rush immunotherapy protocols

AIT has been around for more than 100 years to treat symptoms associated with inhaled allergens.[13,14] Treatments typically involve escalating doses of the allergen of concern over time, with goals of inducing tolerance to the allergen. Guideline-based approaches are available for treatment of aeroallergens and stinging insect venom allergy.[11,17] Venom and aero-AIT treatment was initially pioneered by subcutaneous treatment.

Standard subcutaneous immunotherapy (SCIT) treatment options to environmental pollens and stinging insect venom typically consist of serial escalations in allergen dose, starting with very dilute concentrations of the allergen, often on a weekly basis, until maintenance (an undiluted dose) is achieved, whereby treatments are resumed often on a monthly basis. Rush and cluster immunotherapy protocols exist with expedited schedules to reach maintenance.[18] It is unclear whether rush or cluster aeroallergy immunotherapy SCIT protocols carry a risk of provoking more anaphylactic reactions and an increased need for systemic corticosteroid use. Accelerated protocols in venom immunotherapy (VIT) do not seem associated with an increased anaphylaxis risk.[11]

In the United States, sublingual immunotherapy (SLIT) has recently been Food and Drug Administration approved for grass (Grastek [Merck, Whitehouse Station, NJ] and Oralair [Stallergenes S.A., Antony, France]) and ragweed (Ragwitek [Merck, Whitehouse Station, NJ]), with more options undergoing clinical trials. In Europe and Australia, sublingual therapy has been used for many years.

Food immunotherapy treatment options are evolving, with multiple studies currently being conducted to demonstrate safety and efficacy. Food allergy treatment modalities currently under investigation include Viaskin (DBV Technologies, Bagneux, France), a food allergy patch, and CODIT (Aimmune, Brisbane, CA), an oral immunotherapy food capsule to food(s) with or without omalizumab. SCIT is not approved in food allergy treatment due to an increased risk of anaphylaxis.

PROGNOSIS

- Generally good, but carries a small risk of anaphylaxis
- Allergen immunotherapy requires a compliant and motivated patient
- Treatment of underlying comorbid conditions helps improve response.
- Allergy symptoms usually worsen without treatment.

Studies demonstrate immunotherapy provides benefit for allergic rhinitis, allergic asthma, eczema, and stinging insect venom allergy, with emerging data suggesting benefit for food allergy.[11,17,19–21] Immunotherapy benefits tend to improve with time on treatment. Multiple studies have identified that aero-AIT prevents asthma,[22,23] minimizes symptoms associated with allergen exposure, improves quality of life, and has the potential for beneficial effects on sleep, which may improve productivity at school and/or work.[17,24–27] Additionally, immunotherapy can prevent life-threatening allergic reactions to stinging insects[11] and emerging data are accumulating to suggest the same with food immunotherapy.[19] Despite this, compliance is often poor.[28–31]

A German national health insurance beneficiaries database with a cohort of 118,754 patients demonstrated that among the 2431 (2%) patients treated with immunotherapy in 2006, observed over a 5-year period from 2007 to 2012, and compared with the cohort who did not receive AIT over the same time, AIT was associated with a lower incidence of asthma (relative risk, 0.60; 95% CI, 0.42–0.84).[23]

Variability in response patterns tends to relate to duration of treatment and optimal allergen dosing. Support should be given to increase compliance, with advice to patients on potential side effects and management, assessment of patient motivation, and communication on a regular basis to review treatment response and side effects and to address any fears/concerns associated with treatment.

AIT should be continued for a minimum of 3 years. Studies suggest no additional benefit for treatment beyond 5 years.[32] Individuals with severe systemic allergic reactions to venom might still be in danger on resting, despite 5 years of treatment, and require indefinite VIT treatment.[11] National databases on patient compliance suggest completion of 3 years of AIT is challenging. In a German national database comprising 85,241 patients receiving SCIT to pollen or dust mites and 706 patients receiving pollen SLIT, compliance for 3 years was low, but higher in perennial SCIT at 60% versus 27% for preseasonally administered SCIT; with an overall prescription fill of 42% combined for pollen and 45% combined percent for mites. SLIT compliance was lowest, with 16% of patients completing 3 years of therapy.[28] A Dutch database of 6486 patients, comprising 2796 SCIT-treated and 3690 SLIT-treated patients, demonstrated 18% of the entire group reached 3 years of therapy, of which 23% were SCIT treated and 7% were SLIT treated, respectively.[29] Median SCIT duration was 1.7 years' duration and SLIT was 0.6 years' duration.[29] Studies suggest SLIT compliance success rates are dependent on patient personal motivation.[33]

For subjects who do complete treatment, SCIT is demonstrated efficacious for birch, mountain cedar, grass, ragweed, *Parietaria*, dog, cat, molds *Cladosporium* and *Alternaria*, cockroach, and house dust mites.[17,34–36] Benefits include improved quality of life and decreased medication requirements. Both SLIT and SCIT are cost effective versus pharmacologic management.[34,37–39]

In a Cochrane meta-analysis assessing SLIT asthma, there was not enough evidence to prove efficacy in asthma.[40] Most studies, however, assessed subjects with mild or intermittent asthma and most studies lacked outcome data from validated asthma symptom/quality-of-life questionnaires and medication scores.

Food oral immunotherapy studies suggest benefit. Oral immunotherapy looks promising in peanut, milk, and egg.[41] Food SLIT and food patch studies also look promising.[41,42]

CLINICAL MANAGEMENT

- Concurrent comorbid condition management (both allergic and nonallergic) is important during immunotherapy treatment.
- Asthma should be stable during immunotherapy.
- Patient selection is important.
- Immunotherapy is safe in pregnancy, but dose escalation should not be performed.

AIT improves atopic eczema, allergic rhinitis, allergic asthma, and stinging insect venom allergy. Evidence is increasing for food allergy immunotherapy benefits as well.

The rate of symptom improvement while on immunotherapy can be highly variable, likely due to patient comorbid conditions, patient age, geographic environmental exposures, genetic variability, and compliance.[43] During immunotherapy treatment, concurrent management of comorbid conditions should be implemented per published guidelines. Specifically, comorbid conditions, such as obesity, second-hand tobacco smoke/pollution exposure, and review of patient specific factors, such as gender, age, diet, exercise, and number of allergen triggers (as a correlate to severity), may have an impact on treatment response patterns and outcomes.[44–47] In general, 3 years of immunotherapy have been identified as an important milestone for benefit persistence beyond completion of therapy. More than 5 years of immunotherapy is not thought to provide additional benefit, with the exception of severe venom-allergic individuals, who may require indefinite VIT.[11]

AIT is safe in pregnancy and can be continued at the level achieved on becoming pregnant.[17] Up-dosing should not be performed during pregnancy because increases in immunotherapy dosing can carry the risk of anaphylaxis. Ideally, pregnancy is achieved while on maintenance immunotherapy or initiated in the postpartum period. Contraindications to immunotherapy include noncompliance, unstable asthma, significant cardiovascular disease posing a risk to resuscitation, and anaphylaxis treatment with epinephrine. β-Blocker use is a relative contraindication to immunotherapy due to the potential to negate epinephrine anaphylaxis treatment. VIT treatment failure risk factors include honeybee VIT-induced systemic allergic reaction, mastocytosis, and angiotensin-converting enzyme use.[48]

DISEASE COMPLICATIONS

- Safe when performed by an allergy/immunology specialist
- Unstable asthma is a major risk factor.
- Anaphylaxis and eosinophilic esophagitis in food immunotherapy

Local reactions to immunotherapy are common and include itch, swelling and pain at the treatment site. Local reactions can be treated with supportive care, including ice packs in the first 48 hours to decrease swelling, pretreatment/cotreatment with antihistamines, and heat packs after 48 hours. Systemic reactions to immunotherapy are rare but can be fatal.[17] Hence, the physician administering immunotherapy should discuss the risks and benefits of treatment with patients and provide information on warning signs associated with anaphylaxis. This information should be documented in a patient's medical record and informed consent should be obtained. A majority of systemic reactions to immunotherapy occur within the first 30 minutes after treatment. Hence, patients should be monitored for 30 minutes after treatment and personnel trained in anaphylaxis management and resuscitation should be present during the observation period.

SLIT is approved for home use. Grass SLIT (Grastek) is approved in ages 5 to 65. Ragwitek is approved for ages 18 to 65. The first dose is administered in a physician's office with a 30-minute observation period, 12 weeks before the expected start of the respective allergy season and continued for up to 3 years. Patients should be prescribed an autoinjectable epinephrine at the time of treatment. Severe or uncontrolled asthma, a history of eosinophilic esophagitis, and history of anaphylaxis to SLIT are contraindications to treatment. Oralair, an allergy SLIT tablet, is approved for ages 10 to 65 and comes in 2 doses. Treatment should be initiated 16 weeks before the expected start of grass season and given coseasonally for up to 3 years. The first dose is given in the clinic and subsequent doses are given at home.

Food immunotherapy is in different stages of investigation and treatment modalities. Oral immunotherapy carries the risk of anaphylaxis. Hence, clinical trials evaluating this therapy prescribe autoinjectable epinephrine to subjects undergoing food allergy immunotherapy. In addition to anaphylaxis, potential side effects include emesis, aspiration, abdominal pain, nausea, diarrhea, respiratory symptoms, cardiovascular symptoms, throat swelling, respiratory symptoms, and skin symptoms. It is unclear if eosinophilic esophagitis is a rare potential side effect of food oral immunotherapy, and many clinical trials are screening for this condition prior to, during, and after food immunotherapy trials.[49]

SUMMARY

AIT is a safe, cost-effective method for treating many allergic conditions. AIT may be lifesaving in VIT and in food allergy and AIT can prevent the development and/or progression of asthma. Comorbid diseases, such as obesity, gender, age, and triggers, likely alter immunotherapy response patterns. Patient selection is important. In an era trending toward precision medicine, AIT provides a unique opportunity to personalize medical care.[44]

REFERENCES

1. Seidman MD, Gurgel RK, Lin SY, et al. Clinical practice guideline: allergic rhinitis. Otolaryngol Head Neck Surg 2015;152:S1–43.
2. FastStats: Asthma. Centers for Disease Control and Prevention/National Center for Health Statistics: 2014. Summary Health Statistics Tables for U.S. Adults: National Health Interview Survey, 2014. Table A-2. Available at: http://www.cdc.gov/nchs/fastats/asthma.htm. Accessed May 12, 2016.
3. Izquierdo-Dominguez A, Valero AL, Mullol J. Comparative analysis of allergic rhinitis in children and adults. Curr Allergy Asthma Rep 2013;13:142–51.
4. Pajno GB, Nadeau KC, Passalacqua G, et al. The evolution of allergen and non-specific immunotherapy: past achievements, current applications and future outlook. Expert Rev Clin Immunol 2015;11:141–54.
5. Jackson KD, Howie LD, Akinbami LJ. Trends in allergic conditions among children: United States, 1997-2011. NCHS Data Brief 2013;(121):1–8.
6. Mullins RJ, Dear KB, Tang ML. Time trends in Australian hospital anaphylaxis admissions in 1998-1999 to 2011-2012. J Allergy Clin Immunol 2015;136:367–75.
7. Sicherer SH, Sampson HA. Food allergy: Epidemiology, pathogenesis, diagnosis, and treatment. J Allergy Clin Immunol 2014;133:291–307 [quiz: 308].
8. Bunyavanich S, Rifas-Shiman SL, Platts-Mills TA, et al. Peanut allergy prevalence among school-age children in a US cohort not selected for any disease. J Allergy Clin Immunol 2014;134:753–5.
9. Rudders SA, Arias SA, Camargo CA Jr. Trends in hospitalizations for food-induced anaphylaxis in US children, 2000-2009. J Allergy Clin Immunol 2014;134:960–2.e3.
10. Protudjer JL, Jansson SA, Heibert Arnlind M, et al. Household costs associated with objectively diagnosed allergy to staple foods in children and adolescents. J Allergy Clin Immunol Pract 2015;3:68–75.
11. Golden DB, Moffitt J, Nicklas RA, et al. Stinging insect hypersensitivity: a practice parameter update 2011. J Allergy Clin Immunol 2011;127:852–4.e1-23.
12. Tankersley MS, Ledford DK. Stinging insect allergy: state of the art 2015. J Allergy Clin Immunol Pract 2015;3:315–22 [quiz: 323].
13. Noon L, Cantab BC. Prophylactic inoculation against hay fever. Lancet (London, England) 1911;1572–3.
14. Freeman J, Noon L. Further observation on the treatment of hay-fever by hypodermic inoculation of pollen vaccine. Lancet (London, England) 1911;2:814–7.
15. Fujita H, Soyka MB, Akdis M, et al. Mechanisms of allergen-specific immunotherapy. Clin Transl Allergy 2012;2:2.
16. Rael E. The one airway hypothesis, mechanical, physiologic, immunologic, neurologic, or all of the above? Am J Respir Crit Care Med 2015;191:P993.
17. Cox L, Nelson H, Lockey R, et al. Allergen immunotherapy: a practice parameter third update. J Allergy Clin Immunol 2011;127:S1–55.
18. Calabria CW. Accelerated immunotherapy schedules. Curr Allergy asthma Rep 2013;13:389–98.
19. Sampson HA, Aceves S, Bock SA, et al. Food allergy: a practice parameter update-2014. J Allergy Clin Immunol 2014;134:1016–25.e43.

20. Schneider L, Tilles S, Lio P, et al. Atopic dermatitis: a practice parameter update 2012. J Allergy Clin Immunol 2013;131:295–9.e1-27.

21. Zuberbier T, Bachert C, Bousquet PJ, et al. GA(2) LEN/EAACI pocket guide for allergen-specific immunotherapy for allergic rhinitis and asthma. Allergy 2010; 65:1525–30.

22. Jacobsen L, Niggemann B, Dreborg S, et al. Specific immunotherapy has long-term preventive effect of seasonal and perennial asthma: 10-year follow-up on the PAT study. Allergy 2007;62:943–8.

23. Schmitt J, Schwarz K, Stadler E, et al. Allergy immunotherapy for allergic rhinitis effectively prevents asthma: results from a large retrospective cohort study. J Allergy Clin Immunol 2015;136(6):1511–6.

24. Rael E, Lockey RF. Optimal duration of allergen immunotherapy. J Allergy Clin Immunol 2014;134:1218–9.e2.

25. Didier A, Wahn U, Horak F, et al. Five-grass-pollen sublingual immunotherapy tablet for the treatment of grass-pollen-induced allergic rhinoconjunctivitis: 5 years of experience. Expert Rev Clin Immunol 2014;10:1309–24.

26. Didier A, Malling HJ, Worm M, et al. Post-treatment efficacy of discontinuous treatment with 300IR 5-grass pollen sublingual tablet in adults with grass pollen-induced allergic rhinoconjunctivitis. Clin Exp Allergy 2013;43:568–77.

27. Durham SR, Emminger W, Kapp A, et al. SQ-standardized sublingual grass immunotherapy: confirmation of disease modification 2 years after 3 years of treatment in a randomized trial. J Allergy Clin Immunol 2012;129:717–25.e5.

28. Egert-Schmidt AM, Kolbe JM, Mussler S, et al. Patients' compliance with different administration routes for allergen immunotherapy in Germany. Patient Prefer Adherence 2014;8:1475–81.

29. Kiel MA, Roder E, Gerth van Wijk R, et al. Real-life compliance and persistence among users of subcutaneous and sublingual allergen immunotherapy. J Allergy Clin Immunol 2013;132:353–60.e2.

30. Stokes SC, Quinn JM, Sacha JJ, et al. Adherence to imported fire ant subcutaneous immunotherapy. Ann Allergy Asthma Immunol 2013;110:165–7.

31. Bokanovic D, Aberer W, Griesbacher A, et al. Prevalence of hymenoptera venom allergy and poor adherence to immunotherapy in Austria. Allergy 2011;66:1395–6.

32. Golden DB. Long-term outcome after venom immunotherapy. Curr Opin Allergy Clin Immunol 2010;10:337–41.

33. Antico A. Long-term adherence to sublingual therapy: literature review and suggestions for management strategies based on patients' needs and preferences. Clin Exp Allergy 2014;44:1314–26.

34. Jutel M, Agache I, Bonini S, et al. International consensus on allergy immunotherapy. J Allergy Clin Immunol 2015;136:556–68.

35. Tao L, Shi B, Shi G, et al. Efficacy of sublingual immunotherapy for allergic asthma: retrospective meta-analysis of randomized, double-blind and placebo-controlled trials. Clin Respir J 2014;8:192–205.

36. Incorvaia C, Di Rienzo A, Celani C, et al. Treating allergic rhinitis by sublingual immunotherapy: a review. Ann Ist Super Sanita 2012;48:172–6 .

37. Cox L. Allergy immunotherapy in reducing healthcare cost. Curr Opin Otolaryngol Head Neck Surg 2015;23:247–54.

38. Meadows A, Kaambwa B, Novielli N, et al. A systematic review and economic evaluation of subcutaneous and sublingual allergen immunotherapy in adults and children with seasonal allergic rhinitis. Health Technol Assess 2013;17:vi, xi–xiv, 1–322.

39. Dretzke J, Meadows A, Novielli N, et al. Subcutaneous and sublingual immunotherapy for seasonal allergic rhinitis: a systematic review and indirect comparison. J Allergy Clin Immunol 2013;131:1361–6.
40. Normansell R, Kew KM, Bridgman AL. Sublingual immunotherapy for asthma. Cochrane Database Syst Rev 2015;(8):CD011293.
41. Kulis M, Wright BL, Jones SM, et al. Diagnosis, management, and investigational therapies for food allergies. Gastroenterology 2015;148:1132–42.
42. Sato S, Yanagida N, Ogura K, et al. Immunotherapy in food allergy: towards new strategies. Asian Pac J Allergy Immunol 2014;32:195–202.
43. Rael E. Are environmental factors more important in asthma than genetic factors? J Allergy Clin Immunol 2014;133:AB241.
44. Rael E, Shah P. Asthma phenotype triggers correlate with clinical outcome. Intern Med J 2012;42:11–2.
45. Rael E. Obesity correlates with asthma risk. Am J Respir Crit Care Med 2015;191: A4328.
46. Henao M, Song E, Rosenberg J, et al. Air pollution correlates with ACQ scores. J Allergy Clin Immunol 2015;135:AB108.
47. Gleeson P, Rael E. Association between asthma control and body mass index in asthmatics. Ann Allergy Asthma Immunol 2014;113(5):P68.
48. Rueff F, Vos B, Oude Elberink J, et al. Predictors of clinical effectiveness of Hymenoptera venom immunotherapy. Clin Exp Allergy 2014;44:736–46.
49. Lucendo AJ, Arias A, Tenias JM. Relation between eosinophilic esophagitis and oral immunotherapy for food allergy: a systematic review with meta-analysis. Ann Allergy Asthma Immunol 2014;113:624–9.

Eosinophilic Disorders of the Gastrointestinal Tract

Samiullah, MD[a],*, Hadi Bhurgri, MD[b], Umair Sohail, MD[c]

KEYWORDS

- Eosinophilic gastrointestinal disorder (EGID) • Eosinophilic esophagitis
- Eosinophilic gastroenteritis • Eosinophilic colitis

KEY POINTS

- Eosinophilic gastrointestinal (GI) disorders are a spectrum of disorders marked by eosinophilic infiltration of mucosa without any known cause for eosinophilia.
- Eosinophilic GI disorders can present with variety of symptoms, ranging from anemia, diarrhea, and malabsorption to obstruction and perforation.
- Incidence of eosinophilic esophagitis (EoE) has been increasing over past the 2 decades and is marked by a chronic relapsing course.
- Eosinophilic colitis (EC) can present as infantile or adult form, managed by dietary and pharmacologic therapy, with infantile form running a more benign course.

EOSINOPHILIC GASTROINTESTINAL DISORDERS

GI eosinophilia can be seen in variety of disorders. When there is no established cause of GI eosinophilia, the disorder is termed a primary eosinophilic GI disorder (EGID). The entire GI tract from esophagus to colon can be affected. This group of disorders includes EoE, gastroenteritis, and less frequently colitis.[1] Causes of GI eosinophilia are summarized in **Box 1**.[2,3]

EOSINOPHILIC ESOPHAGITIS
Introduction

EoE is described as a constellation of esophageal dysfunction, notably dysphagia, with an eosinophil-predominant infiltrate seen on histology. Other causes of esophageal eosinophilia have to be ruled out.[4]

EoE became increasingly recognized as an entity in the 1990s, although first described in 1978.[5] Given recent interest and possibly increasing incidence, much research has been done over the past 2 decades. Diagnostic controversy exists

[a] Division of Gastroenterology, University of Missouri, 1 Hospital Drive, Columbia, MO 65212, USA; [b] Rutgers University, New Jersey Medical School, 150 Bergen Street, I-248, Newark, NJ 07103, USA; [c] Division of Gastroenterology-Hepatology, University of Missouri, 1 Hospital Drive, Columbia, MO 65212, USA
* Corresponding author.
E-mail address: samiullah.nabi@gmail.com

Prim Care Clin Office Pract 43 (2016) 495–504
http://dx.doi.org/10.1016/j.pop.2016.04.003
0095-4543/16/$ – see front matter © 2016 Elsevier Inc. All rights reserved.
primarycare.theclinics.com

Box 1
Causes of gastrointestinal eosinophilia

Inflammatory bowel disease

Parasites
  Hookworms (*Ancylostoma caninum, Necator americanus*)
  Pinworms (*Enterobius vermicularis*)
  Eustoma rotundatum
  Ascaris lumbricoides
  Trichuris trichiura

Medications
  Nonsteroidal anti-inflammatory drugs
  Enalapril
  Clozapine
  Carbamazepine
  Rifampin
  Gold salts

Malignancy
  Leukemia
  Hodgkin disease
  Graft-versus-host disease

Autoimmune
  Churg-Strauss syndrome
  Hyper-IgE syndrome
  Hypereosinophilic syndrome
  Polyarteritis nodosa

Data from Hurrell JM, Genta RM, Melton SD. Histopathologic diagnosis of eosinophilic conditions in the gastrointestinal tract. Adv Anat Pathol 2011;18(5):335–48; and Liacouras CA. Eosinophilic gastrointestinal disorders. Practical Gastroenterol 2007;31:53–66.

over the determination of the thresholds for eosinophilia and is compounded by the overall varying symptomatology of EoE. Not all esophageal eosinophilia is classified as EoE. A distinction must be made with the entity proton-pump inhibitor (PPI) responsive esophageal eosinophilia (PPI-REE) and gastroesophageal reflux disease (GERD), in which acid exposure may induce an eosinophilic infiltrate. This usually resolves by prescribing high dose proton pump inhibitors for 8 weeks.[4,6]

EoE has a bimodal distribution. It affects children and is also manifested during the third and fourth decades of life. It predominantly affects boys and men (3:1 male-to-female ratio), and frequently affects non-Hispanic whites. The incidence seems to be increasing. It is frequently a chronic condition with high rates of relapse seen on discontinuing treatment.

The first consensus guidelines were formulated in 2007, with updates from the International Gastrointestinal Eosinophil Researchers (TIGERS) Summary of 2011.[6] The most recent practice guidelines are from the American College of Gastroenterology from 2015.[4]

Basic Pathophysiology

The pathogenesis of EoE involves a complex interplay of genetic, dietary, and environmental factors, causing an eosinophilic infiltrate in the esophageal mucosa, which is normally devoid of eosinophils.[7,8] The exact immune-mediated mechanisms for the esophageal infiltrate are not known and could be immunoglobulin E (IgE) mediated and also delayed type 2 helper T cell (T_H2) responses. Certain interleukins (ILs), notably IL-5, IL-13, and IL-15 expression, are associated with EoE. Dietary allergens are known to play a role in this antigen/immune condition. A positive family history is also frequently observed in patients, and some susceptibility genes have been identified.[8] Genetic testing is available commercially, but routine use in clinical practice has not been established.[9]

Clinical Presentation

The typical clinical presentation involves a young man in his 30s who complains of dysphagia, although a variety of upper GI symptoms may exist. Food impactions are common and may be the presenting symptom.[10] Other symptoms include reflux, retrosternal pain, and abdominal pain in adults. Careful history taking is essential, because patients may have developed compensatory strategies, for example, excessively washing food down with liquids, eating very slowly, or avoidance of certain foods like meat and breads.[11]

For pediatric age groups, symptoms are similar but expression of symptoms depends on age. In addition there may be an aversion of food, regurgitation, or vomiting.[12]

An association is noted with atopy in general, and a high frequency of asthma, eczema, and allergic rhinosinusitis is seen in patients with EoE. Although peripheral eosinophilia may be seen in EoE, it is not considered diagnostic, and specifically esophageal mucosal eosinophilia must be established.

Diagnosis

Several clinical conditions are associated with esophageal eosinophilia and esophageal dysfunction. The notable distinction that has to be made is GERD. A common presentation of EoE is reflux. Acid exposure from GERD itself can induce an eosinophilic infiltrate in the esophagus, although that resolves after PPI therapy. It is essential that biopsies be obtained after treatment with PPIs for a 2-month period, to exclude so called PPI-REE.[4]

Other differential diagnoses need to be considered depending on specific presenting symptoms. For patients who present with dysphagia and food impactions, congenital rings, strictures, and achalasia need to be considered. Other conditions, such as infectious esophagitis, drug hypersensitivity, hypereosinophilic syndromes, Crohn's disease, autoimmune disorders, and celiac disease should be ruled out.

A diagnosis of EoE begins with a careful history specifically eliciting esophageal dysfunction, including but not limited to dysphagia, reflux, retrosternal pain, and a history of food impactions.

Endoscopic findings include so-called feline esophagus, which refers to mucosal rings or a corrugated appearance seen on endoscopy. Other endoscopic findings include plaques, mucosal edema, decreased vascularity, narrowing, and furrows. A reliable diagnosis can, however, be made only with histology, and endoscopic appearance alone is not sufficient for diagnosis.

Esophageal biopsies must demonstrate mucosal eosinophilia of at least 15 per high-power field (HPF), although in true EoE, it typically exceeds 20 per HPF. PPI-REE can also present with greater than 15 eosinophils per HPF. Biopsies must be obtained from the proximal and distal esophagus and typically at least 6 biopsies are suggested to maximize the yield.[13] The esophageal eosinophilia must persist after a 2-month trial of PPI treatment, and other causes of secondary eosinophilia must be ruled out. Also, although not essential for diagnosing EoE, the eosinophilic infiltrate should respond to dietary restriction and topical steroids.

Management

In general, EoE is a chronic disorder, with frequent relapses after discontinuing treatment, and patients need to be counseled regarding the nature of the disease. A multidisciplinary approach is preferred in conjunction with gastroenterologist, allergist/immunologist and dieticians.

Treatment options include dietary restriction, topical steroids, and, in cases of severe strictures or a narrow caliber esophagus, endoscopic dilation. Systemic steroids, such as prednisone, typically have no role in the treatment of EoE given a nonfavorable risk/benefit profile. Patients should be monitored for oral candidiasis while on topical steroids.

Fluticasone and budesonide have been studied for topical corticosteroid therapy. Swallowed, rather than inhaled, fluticasone is used with a multidose inhaler preparation. The most recent American College of Gastroenterology guidelines suggest swallowed fluticasone at a dose of 88 μg/d to 440 μg/d in divided doses for children and 880 μg/d to 1760 μg/d in divided doses for adults.[4,14]

Budesonide is used in the form of swallowed nebulizer preparations and also a viscous liquid slurry. A dose of 1 mg/d is suggested in children and 2 mg/d in adults in divided doses. The liquid preparation is useful in the pediatric population and prepared by mixing 1 mg/2 mL of aqueous budesonide with 5 g of sucralose.[15]

Dietary restriction treatment consists of 3 main approaches, and in general is better studied in children, with the philosophy of potentially avoiding long-term pharmaco-logic therapy.[16] They consist of an elemental diet consisting of amino acid–based formulas, which eliminates all potential food allergens; a testing guided food elimination diet; and an empiric 6-food elimination diet, which eliminates soy, egg, milk, wheat, nuts, and seafood from the diet (agents that are known triggers of EoE). Elimination guided by skin prick or patch testing has also been used, although there is controversy over whether cutaneous allergy testing can effectively predict EoE triggers in adults. Another approach is predicting triggers based on food reintroduction after elimination diet initiation. With strict adherence, response has been noted for several years; however, as with pharmacologic treatment, recurrence of EoE is seen with nonadherence.[17–19]

Endoscopic treatment is generally reserved for patients with severe disease that is refractory to the therapies discussed previously and in whom significant stenosis is present. It involves gradual endoscopic dilation. Earlier studies of dilation reported very high rates of complications, including perforations, although more recent evidence suggests that in experienced hands the complications are much lower than originally anticipated. It is recommended that this be performed at high-volume tertiary centers given potential complications.[20]

EOSINOPHILIC GASTROENTERITIS
Introduction

Eosinophilic gastroenteritis (EG) is an inflammatory disorder characterized by eosinophilic infiltration of the stomach and small intestine. EG is seen in higher socioeconomic classes, with a prevalence of 22 to 28 per 100,000 persons in the United States.[21] It affects both adults and children, typically affecting adults in their third to fifth decades. The disease has been reportedly more prevalent in patients with seasonal allergies, food sensitivities, eczema, allergic rhinitis, and asthma.[22]

Basic Pathophysiology

The exact pathogenesis of EG is not well understood. Several studies have suggested an allergic component.[23] In allergic EG patients, a population of IL-5 expressing food allergen–specific T_H2 cells have been identified. This suggests that food exposure activates and drives the differentiation of T_H2 cells leading to recruitment of eosinophils in the GI tract. Eosinophils cause local inflammation, leading to intestinal epithelial damage by release of eosinophilic major basic protein, a cytotoxic cationic protein.[24] Patients with EGID may have elevated serum IgE levels.[25] The elevated levels of serum IgE suggest that atopy may be involved in the pathogenesis of the disease.[26]

Clinical Presentation

Approximately one-half of patients with EG have a history of allergic disorders, including eczema, asthma, defined food allergies, or rhinitis. The disease often waxes and wanes in severity. The clinical features of eosinophilic disorders depend on the extent of the disease and degree of involvement of GI wall layers with eosinophilic infiltrates. It may be limited to the mucosa or penetrate deep into muscularis layer and serosa.

Patients with superficial involvement present with abdominal pain, nausea, vomiting, and diarrhea.[23] Patients with extensive involvement of small bowel mucosa may have malabsorption, protein-losing enteropathy, failure to thrive, and weight loss. The eosinophilic infiltration of the deep layers of the GI tract usually leads to wall thickening and impaired motility. As a result, patients usually present with symptoms of intestinal obstruction, including nausea, vomiting, and abdominal distention.[23] In severe cases, deeper eosinophilic infiltration can lead to perforation, gastric outlet obstruction, or small bowel obstruction. When the disease penetrates the subserosal layers, it can present with eosinophilic ascites.

Diagnosis

EG should be suspected in patients who present with complaints of abdominal pain, nausea, vomiting, early satiety, diarrhea, weight loss, or ascites associated with peripheral eosinophilia (eosinophil count >500/µL in the peripheral blood). A detailed history of seasonal allergies, food allergics or food intolerance, and other allergic conditions, such as asthma and eczema, should be obtained. Dietary history should include the ingestion of raw or undercooked meat and history of residence in or recent travel to parasite endemic areas.

Laboratory evaluation reveals an elevated eosinophil count (5%–35% or average 1000 cells/µL) in 80% of cases. The erythrocyte sedimentation rate and C-reactive protein levels can be elevated in up to 20% of cases.[23,27] Patients with severe mucosal EG present with malabsorption and protein-losing enteropathy, manifesting as hypoalbuminemia. Iron deficiency anemia is seen due to both malabsorption and blood loss.[28,29] Serum IgE levels are usually elevated, especially in children. Stool studies and serologic studies should be performed to exclude a parasitic infection.

Radiologically, EG shows nodular thickening of the folds in distal stomach and proximal small intestine. Imaging in patients with muscular involvement may reveal irregular luminal narrowing, especially in the distal antrum and proximal small bowel. All these findings are neither sensitive nor specific for EG, however, because similar thickening of GI wall may be seen in Ménétrier disease, lymphoma, Crohn's disease, and granulomatous disease.[26]

The endoscopic features of EG are nonspecific, including erythematous, friable, nodular, and occasional ulcerative changes. Eosinophilic infiltrates are usually patchy in distribution and may coexist with normal mucosal architecture; therefore, multiple biopsies are required to avoid missing the diagnosis.[26] A diagnosis of mucosal EG is established by the presence of more than the number of expected eosinophils on microscopic examination of biopsy specimens of the GI tract.[28,30] There is no defined cutoff for the number of eosinophils per HPF to diagnose EG. The histologic slides should be confirmed by an experienced GI pathologist to assess if the number of eosinophils is more than expected for a particular area. Negative mucosal biopsies do not definitively rule out the disease because patients with muscular and subserosal involvement may have normal mucosal biopsies. In these cases, a laparoscopic full-thickness biopsy is necessary to establish the diagnosis.

Management

There is a dearth of evidence pertaining to the treatment of EG. The treatment is based on severity of symptoms. It is useful to look for specific food allergies, because an elimination diet may be successful in improvement of the symptoms. The 6-food elimination diet is the most commonly used empiric elimination diet for EG. Specific foods that are avoided in the 6-food elimination diet include soy, wheat, egg, milk, peanut/tree nuts, and seafood.[17]

Dietary therapy should be pursued in motivated patients and under the guidance of a dietitian trained in eosinophilic GI disorders. If a history of environmental allergens is identified, these should be treated in conjunction with the diet. The role of the dietician includes patient education on the use of antigen-free foods, allergen avoidance, and food suggestions to ensure a nutritionally adequate diet. In patients with peripheral eosinophilia, after being on elimination diet, it is suggested to recheck the peripheral eosinophil count. A reduction of more than 50% in the eosinophil count may be considered a response. This approach cannot be used, however, in patients with normal eosinophil counts at the onset of treatment. If the dietary changes are successful at reducing symptoms and either peripheral or tissue eosinophilia, foods can be reintroduced gradually in a systematic fashion from least allergenic to most allergenic.

In cases of dietary elimination not improving the symptoms, a trial of corticosteroids should be given. The evidence to support the use of steroids is based on limited data from small case series.[22,26] Glucocorticoids can be used as systemic or topical agents to achieve improvement in symptoms. Systemic steroids are used for acute exacerbations, whereas topical steroids are used to provide long-term relief in cases of dietary restrictions not being feasible or having failed to improve the symptoms.[31] The improvement in symptoms usually occurs within 2 weeks regardless of the extent of bowel layer involvement. Steroids should be tapered over 2 weeks after improvement of symptoms. Some patients, however, may require a prolonged course of therapy with steroids for up to several months to achieve complete resolution of symptoms. In patients who experience recurrent symptoms during or immediately after the prednisone taper, long-term, low-dose maintenance therapy with prednisone is needed.[30] In patients with distal ileal disease, controlled ileal release capsules (budesonide) may prove an effective therapy.

There are several case reports and case series describing use of alternate agents for control of symptoms. These agents differ in their mechanism of action to help decrease the inflammation. One of the approaches includes the use of cromolyn as a steroid-sparing agent. Cromolyn works by preventing the release of mast cell mediators, including histamine, platelet-activating factor, and leukotriene, and is also thought to reduce absorption of antigens by the small intestine. Montelukast, a competitive cysteinyl leukotriene-1 receptor antagonist, has also been used as a treatment of EG. Friesen and colleagues[32] conducted a double-blind, randomized, placebo-controlled, crossover study of montelukast therapy. In this study, the patients received either montelukast (10 mg) or an identical placebo once daily and were evaluated on day 14 for symptomatic and biochemical responses. A positive clinical result was seen in 62.1% of patients receiving montelukast compared with 32.4% on placebo ($P<.02$).

IL-5 is an important inflammatory marker involved in the development, differentiation, mobilization, and activation of eosinophils. Prussin and colleagues[33] treated 4 patients with EG with a single dose of humanized anti–IL-5 monoclonal antibody. The results showed a decrease in peripheral eosinophilia and tissue eosinophilia in 75% of patients. There was minimal improvement, however, in symptoms.

Omalizumab is a humanized therapeutic monoclonal antibody that binds to IgE, thus preventing IgE from activating mast cells and basophils and decreasing the concentration of high-affinity IgE receptors on these cells. Omalizumab has been shown to decrease the eosinophil counts in EG.[34] Controlled, randomized trials to determine the efficacy of these agents, however, are lacking.

EOSINOPHILIC COLITIS
Introduction

EC is a rare disorder and the exact prevalence remains unknown. EC has a bimodal distribution, with high prevalence in neonates and young adults with no gender preference.[35] Common causes of eosinophilia, such as parasites, medications, and inflammatory bowel disease (IBD), need to be ruled out in these patients.

Basic Pathophysiology

Normally, dietary antigens are presented in nonantigenic form to the immune system by enterocytes; however, early on in life, the GI tract may not serve as effective barrier to dietary antigens. This leads to presentation of intact dietary antigens to immune system, triggering an inappropriate immune response against the GI tract.[3] Common foods associated with the infantile form of EC are cow milk and soy protein. Approximately half the patients with EC are exclusively fed breast milk and elimination of cow milk protein from the mother's diet does not always resolve the symptoms, suggesting a role for multiple food allergies.[36,37]

Clinical Presentation

EC can present with a variety of symptoms. Patients commonly present with blood in stool, which may or may not be related to diarrheal illness. The blood often presents as streaks in stool. These patients may present with iron deficiency anemia and protein-losing enteropathy. In disease affecting the deeper layers of colonic wall and serosal involvement intestinal obstruction, intussusception and perforation have also been reported.[36,38] Patients with serosal involvement can present with eosinophilic ascites.

Diagnosis

EC is a diagnosis of exclusion. Colonic eosinophilia can be seen in patients with parasitic infections, malignancies, and patients taking certain medications (**Box 1**). IBD can present with colonic eosinophils. Eosinophils are predominantly seen in patients with Crohn's colitis. Patients with IBD also show evidence of chronic distortion of mucosal architecture on biopsy specimens.

It is important to obtain a travel history and rule out parasitic infections with stool and serologic studies. It is important to ask patients for a complete medication history to rule out medication-induced eosinophilia, especially over-the-counter nonsteroidal anti-inflammatory drugs.

Colonoscopy in EC reveals nonspecific findings of erythema and loss of normal vascular pattern. Histology shows eosinophilic infiltration with well-preserved mucosal architecture. There is no specific cutoff for number of eosinophils per HPF; however a diagnostic value of greater than 20 eosinophils per HPF has been used.[35,37]

Management

The infantile form of EC usually demonstrates a benign course. Symptoms usually resolve after discontinuation of the offending allergen, such as cow milk.[37] For patients who are exclusively breastfed, cow milk protein should be excluded from mother's diet and breastfeeding should be continued.[36]

The management of EC in adults is more challenging than eosinophilic esophagitis or gastroenteritis, and may require treatment with immunosuppressive medications.[37] There are no randomized controlled trials for treatment of EC due to rarity of disease. Parasitic infections should be ruled out by appropriate serologic and stool testing before steroids are initiated because steroids can worsen these conditions. Corticosteroids have shown effective in patients with EC. A response is seen with a 2-week treatment; however, relapse is frequent, leading to steroid dependence. In patients with right-sided disease, budesonide, a synthetic oral corticosteroid, has been shown effective in EGID. Azathioprine or 6 mercaptopurine, montelukast (leukotriene D4 blocker), cromolyn (mast cell stabilizer), mepolizumab (monoclonal antibody against IL-5), and omalizumab (monoclonal antibody against IgE) also have been described in management of EGID.[38,39]

SUMMARY

EGIDs have been increasingly diagnosed over the past few years and have drawn a tremendous amount of interest. A diagnosis of EGID requires exclusion of other known disorders causing GI eosinophilia; hence, it is important to obtain a good history and physical examination. Serologic testing and tissue biopsy specimens remain important for diagnosis of these disorders. Treatment largely consists of alteration of diet and corticosteroids. Novel treatment modalities targeting immune modulation are being investigated and will likely show promising results in the future.

REFERENCES

1. Zuo L, Rothenberg ME. Gastrointestinal eosinophilia. Immunol Allergy Clin N Am 2007;27(3):443–55.
2. Hurrell JM, Genta RM, Melton SD. Histopathologic diagnosis of eosinophilic conditions in the gastrointestinal tract. Adv Anat Pathol 2011;18(5):335–48.
3. Liacouras CA. Eosinophilic gastrointestinal disorders. Pract Gastroenterol 2007; 31:53–66.
4. Dellon ES, Gonsalves N, Hirano I, et al. ACG clinical guideline: evidenced based approach to the diagnosis and management of esophageal eosinophilia and eosinophilic esophagitis (EoE). Am J Gastroenterol 2013;108(5):679–92 [quiz: 93].
5. Landres RT, Kuster GG, Strum WB. Eosinophilic esophagitis in a patient with vigorous achalasia. Gastroenterology 1978;74(6):1298–301.
6. Liacouras CA, Furuta GT, Hirano I, et al. Eosinophilic esophagitis: updated consensus recommendations for children and adults. J Allergy Clin Immunol 2011;128(1):3–20.e6 [quiz: 1–2].
7. Green DJ, Cotton CC, Dellon ES. The role of environmental exposures in the etiology of eosinophilic esophagitis: a systematic review. Mayo Clin Proc 2015; 90(10):1400–10.
8. D'Alessandro A, Esposito D, Pesce M, et al. Eosinophilic esophagitis: from pathophysiology to treatment. World J Gastrointest Pathophysiol 2015;6(4):150–8.

9. Wen T, Stucke EM, Grotjan TM, et al. Molecular diagnosis of eosinophilic esophagitis by gene expression profiling. Gastroenterology 2013;145(6):1289–99.

10. Sperry SL, Crockett SD, Miller CB, et al. Esophageal foreign-body impactions: epidemiology, time trends, and the impact of the increasing prevalence of eosinophilic esophagitis. Gastrointest Endosc 2011;74(5):985–91.

11. Miehlke S. Clinical features of eosinophilic esophagitis. Dig Dis 2014;32(1–2): 61–7.

12. Kapel RC, Miller JK, Torres C, et al. Eosinophilic esophagitis: a prevalent disease in the United States that affects all age groups. Gastroenterology 2008;134(5): 1316–21.

13. Saffari H, Peterson KA, Fang JC, et al. Patchy eosinophil distributions in an esophagectomy specimen from a patient with eosinophilic esophagitis: implications for endoscopic biopsy. J Allergy Clin Immunol 2012;130(3):798–800.

14. Konikoff MR, Noel RJ, Blanchard C, et al. A randomized, double-blind, placebo-controlled trial of fluticasone propionate for pediatric eosinophilic esophagitis. Gastroenterology 2006;131(5):1381–91.

15. Dellon ES, Sheikh A, Speck O, et al. Viscous topical is more effective than nebulized steroid therapy for patients with eosinophilic esophagitis. Gastroenterology 2012;143(2):321–4.e1.

16. Gonsalves N, Kagalwalla AF. Dietary treatment of eosinophilic esophagitis. Gastroenterol Clin North Am 2014;43(2):375–83.

17. Kagalwalla AF, Sentongo TA, Ritz S, et al. Effect of six-food elimination diet on clinical and histologic outcomes in eosinophilic esophagitis. Clin Gastroenterol Hepatol 2006;4(9):1097–102.

18. Gonsalves N, Yang GY, Doerfler B, et al. Elimination diet effectively treats eosinophilic esophagitis in adults, food reintroduction identifies causative factors. Gastroenterology 2012;142(7):1451–9.e1 [quiz: e14–5].

19. Lucendo AJ, Arias A, Gonzalez-Cervera J, et al. Empiric 6-food elimination diet induced and maintained prolonged remission in patients with adult eosinophilic esophagitis: a prospective study on the food cause of the disease. J Allergy Clin Immunol 2013;131(3):797–804.

20. Schoepfer AM, Gonsalves N, Bussmann C, et al. Esophageal dilation in eosinophilic esophagitis: effectiveness, safety, and impact on the underlying inflammation. Am J Gastroenterol 2010;105(5):1062–70.

21. Spergel JM, Book WM, Mays E, et al. Variation in prevalence, diagnostic criteria, and initial management options for eosinophilic gastrointestinal diseases in the United States. J Pediatr Gastroenterol Nutr 2011;52(3):300–6.

22. von Wattenwyl F, Zimmermann A, Netzer P. Synchronous first manifestation of an idiopathic eosinophilic gastroenteritis and bronchial asthma. Eur J Gastroenterol Hepatol 2001;13(6):721–5.

23. Talley NJ, Shorter RG, Phillips SF, et al. Eosinophilic gastroenteritis: a clinicopathological study of patients with disease of the mucosa, muscle layer, and subserosal tissues. Gut 1990;31(1):54–8.

24. Talley NJ, Kephart GM, McGovern TW, et al. Deposition of eosinophil granule major basic protein in eosinophilic gastroenteritis and celiac disease. Gastroenterology 1992;103(1):137–45.

25. Caldwell JH, Tennenbaum JI, Bronstein HA. Serum IgE in eosinophilic gastroenteritis. Response to intestinal challenge in two cases. N Engl J Med 1975;292(26): 1388–90.

26. Chen MJ, Chu CH, Lin SC, et al. Eosinophilic gastroenteritis: clinical experience with 15 patients. World J Gastroenterol 2003;9(12):2813–6.

27. Cello JP. Eosinophilic gastroenteritis–a complex disease entity. Am J Med 1979; 67(6):1097–104.
28. Katz AJ, Goldman H, Grand RJ. Gastric mucosal biopsy in eosinophilic (allergic) gastroenteritis. Gastroenterology 1977;73(4 Pt 1):705–9.
29. Klein NC, Hargrove RL, Sleisenger MH, et al. Eosinophilic gastroenteritis. Medicine 1970;49(4):299–319.
30. Lee CM, Changchien CS, Chen PC, et al. Eosinophilic gastroenteritis: 10 years experience. Am J Gastroenterol 1993;88(1):70–4.
31. Jawairia M, Shahzad G, Mustacchia P. Eosinophilic gastrointestinal diseases: review and update. ISRN Gastroenterol 2012;2012:463689.
32. Friesen CA, Kearns GL, Andre L, et al. Clinical efficacy and pharmacokinetics of montelukast in dyspeptic children with duodenal eosinophilia. J Pediatr Gastroenterol Nutr 2004;38(3):343–51.
33. Prussin C, James SP, Huber MM, et al. Pilot study of anti IL 5 in eosinophilic gastroenteritis. J Allergy Clin Immunol 2003;111(1):S275.
34. Foroughi S, Foster B, Kim N, et al. Anti-IgE treatment of eosinophil-associated gastrointestinal disorders. J Allergy Clin Immunol 2007;120(3):594–601.
35. Okpara N, Aswad B, Baffy G. Eosinophilic colitis. World J Gastroenterol 2009; 15(24):2975–9.
36. Lozinsky AC, Morais MB. Eosinophilic colitis in infants. J Pediatr 2014;90(1): 16–21.
37. Rothenberg ME. Eosinophilic gastrointestinal disorders (EGID). J Allergy Clin Immunol 2004;113(1):11–28 [quiz: 9].
38. Alfadda AA, Storr MA, Shaffer EA. Eosinophilic colitis: epidemiology, clinical features, and current management. Therap Adv Gastroenterol 2011;4(5):301–9.
39. Gaertner WB, Macdonald JE, Kwaan MR, et al. Eosinophilic colitis: University of Minnesota experience and literature review. Gastroenterol Res Pract 2011;2011: 857508.

Mastocytosis

Ayesha Abid, MD*, Michael A. Malone, MD,
Katherine Curci, PhD, NP

KEYWORDS

- Masocytosis • Update • Review • Pathophysiology • Diagnosis • Treatment
- Cutaneous mastocytosis • Systemic mastocytosis

KEY POINTS

- Mastocytosis is a rare disease, characterized by excessive production of mast cells that accumulate in the skin, bone marrow, and other visceral organs.
- The prevalence of mastocytosis is estimated to be 1 in 60,000 in the United States; children tend to have benign forms of mastocytosis, whereas adults may develop aggressive disease.
- The most common mutation is in the C-kit gene, which causes increased proliferation of mast cells; other causes exist but are less frequent.
- Clinical presentation of mastocytosis is variable, often based on the type of mastocytosis, but in all types of mastocytosis there seems to be an increase in the risk of anaphylaxis; patients may present with skin lesions, flushing, diarrhea, lymphadenopathy, hepatosplenomegaly, osteoporosis, and recurrent anaphylaxis.
- For systemic mastocytosis (SM), the preferred method of diagnosing is via bone marrow biopsy.

INTRODUCTION

Mastocytosis is a rare disease, characterized by excessive production of mast cells that accumulate in the skin, bone marrow, and other visceral organs.[1] In a majority of cases, the disorder is due to a nonhereditary somatic mutation in the KIT gene, which leads to heightened proliferation and activation of morphologically and clinically abnormal mast cells.[2] Mast cell activation results in release of mediators by degranulation, and synthesis of lipids and proteins.[3] These mediators are responsible for the clinical manifestations, which include pruritus, flushing, diarrhea, headaches, and life-threatening anaphylaxis.[3] The World Health Organization (WHO) has classified mastocytosis into 7 categories. Broadly, it can be divided into cutaneous mastocytosis (CM) and SM. CM is relatively benign and affects the skin whereas SM involves an extracutaneous organ and has aggressive potential.[4] The most common form of CM is urticarial pigmentosa.[5] SM is subclassified into indolent SM (ISM), associated

Department of Family and Community Medicine, Penn State Milton S. Hershey Medical Center, 500 University Drive, Hershey, PA 17033, USA
* Corresponding author.
E-mail address: aabid@hmc.psu.edu

Prim Care Clin Office Pract 43 (2016) 505–518
http://dx.doi.org/10.1016/j.pop.2016.04.007
0095-4543/16/$ – see front matter © 2016 Elsevier Inc. All rights reserved.
primarycare.theclinics.com

clonal hematologic non–mast cell lineage disease (AHNMD), aggressive SM (ASM), and mast cell leukemia (MCL) (**Table 1**).

EPIDEMIOLOGY

The prevalence of mastocytosis is estimated to be 1 in 60,000 in the United States. The disease occurs in both children and adults. Children tend to have benign forms of mastocytosis, whereas adults may develop aggressive disease. The true number of cases of mastocytosis is unknown.[1] Its prevalence is estimated to be 1 in 60,000 and incidence 0.5 to 1 per 100,000 per year in the United States.[6] Mastocytosis is a disease of both children and adults, with equal male and female prevalence.[7] A majority of patients are children and are typically affected by CM forms, which carry an excellent prognosis.[8] In many children, symptoms regress spontaneously by puberty.[8] Adults are much more likely to have urticarial pigmentosa and ISM. In adults, the onset of mastocytosis is generally at age 20 to 50 and is diagnosed between 40 and 60 years of age.[3,7] The disease is congenital in approximately 15% to 25% of cases and, in these patients, usually occurs before the age of 2.[3,7,9] In a majority of cases, the disease is spontaneous.[3]

MAST CELL BIOLOGY

Mast cells act as effector cells in allergic and hypersensitivity disorders and are activated through IgE and non-IgE mechanisms. Once activated, they release proinflammatory and vasoactive mediators. Mast cells arise from pluripotent cells in the bone marrow, acquire cytoplasmic granules, and mature in specialized tissues.[1,4,7] They act as sentinels of the innate and adaptive immune system and are abundant in endothelial and mucosal surfaces.[2,6,10,11] Mast cells have a central role in immunomodulation and act as effector cells in allergic and hypersensitivity disorders.[12] Activation and degranulation of mast cells occur through IgE and non-IgE receptor cross-linking.[7,10]

Table 1 World health organization classification of mastocytosis	
CM	• Urticaria pigmentosa or maculopapular CM • DCM • Mastocytoma of skin

SM	• ISM
	  ○ Isolated bone marrow mastocytosis
	  ○ Smoldering SM
	• SM-AHNMD
	  ○ SM with acute myeloid leukemia
	  ○ SM with myelodysplastic syndrome
	  ○ SM with myeloproliferative disorder
	  ○ SM with chronic myelomonocytic leukemia
	  ○ SM with hypereosinophilic syndrome
	• ASM
	  ○ Lymphopathic SM with eosinophilia
	• MCL
	  ○ Classic
	  ○ Aleukemic MCL

MCS	
Extracutaneous mastocytoma	

Data from Valent P, Akin C, Wolfgang S, et al. Mastocytosis: pathology, genetics and current options for therapy. Leuk Lymphoma 2005;46:35–48.

Non-IgE–mediated activation includes hymenoptera stings, foods, drugs, alcohol, physical and emotional stimuli, heat, cold, exercise, ionizing radiation, complement, hormones, and cytokines.[7,13] Pharmacologic agents, such as nonsteroidal anti-inflammatory drugs (NSAIDs), opioids, and muscle relaxants, cause mast cell mediator release, most notable in skin mast cells.[14] When activated, granules within mast cells release histamine, serotonin, heparin, phospholipases, and proteases (ie, tryptase and chymase), prostaglandins, thromboxanes, cytokines, tumor necrosis factor, and growth factors.[7,10–12] Tryptases and chymases account for the bulk of protein release from mast cell secretory granules.[10] Tryptase is produced almost exclusively by mast cells and, therefore, is used as a biological marker of disease.[14]

PATHOPHYSIOLOGY

The most common mutation is in the C-kit gene, which causes increased proliferation of mast cells. Other causes exist but are less frequent (**Table 2**).

CLINICAL MANIFESTATIONS

Clinical presentation of mastocytosis is variable, often based on the type of mastocytosis, but in all types of mastocytosis there seems to be an increase the risk of anaphylaxis. Patients may present with skin lesions, flushing, diarrhea, lymphadenopathy, hepatosplenomegaly, osteoporosis, and recurrent anaphylaxis.[13] Lung and kidney involvement is rare.[3] The most common symptom is pruritus.

Symptoms often vary based on the type of mastocytosis. The clinical manifestations of the disease may be variable, ranging from asymptomatic disease to systemic involvement.[3,6] This depends the extent of mast cell penetration in tissues.[6] CM is due to limited aggregation of mast cells in skin tissues.[10] For CM, common symptoms are itching, swelling, and blistering of the affected skin, particularly when it is rubbed or scratched, and is sometimes associated with abdominal cramping or anaphylaxis.

SM symptoms may be chronic or episodic.[3] In progressive stages of the disease, mast cell end-organ damage causes weight loss and pathologic fractures and ascites may occur.[3,14] The most common trigger of symptoms in SM is stress.[12] Most patients present with classic skin findings and may be diagnosed with urticarial pigmentosa. The absence of skin findings in SM is rare and is correlated with aggressive disease (**Table 3**).[6]

Table 2 Causes of mastocytosis and pathophysiologic effect	
Etiology	**Effect**
C-kit gene mutation	"Activating" mutation → increased productivity → increase in mast cells numbers and activation (SM)
Other mutations: FIP1L1/PDGFRA, JAK2V617F, RAS, TET2 and IgE receptor genes	SM forms: SM-AHNMD, ASM, and MCL
CD2 cell surface antigen expression	CD2-CD58 interaction → infiltration of mast cell in tissue → release of mediators → organ damage → disease sequelae
Failure of mast cell apoptosis	Increase number of mast cells → release of mediators → organ damage → disease sequelae

Data from Refs.[3,7,9,10,15–17]

Table 3
Clinical manifestations of mastocystosis

Organ System	Symptoms/Findings
Constitutional	Fatigue, lethargy, weight loss, chills, weakness, sweats, fever
Skin	Flushing, pruritus, urticaria, hives, angioedema
Neurologic/ psychological	Headaches, trouble concentrating, dizziness, depression, anxiety, sleep disturbances
Respiratory	Anaphylaxis, shortness of breath, wheezing, nasal congestion, nasal pruritus
Cardiovascular	Hypotension, palpitations, tachycardia, syncopal episodes, light-headedness, pericardial effusions
GI	Diarrhea, nausea, vomiting, abdominal pain, bloating, heartburn, peptic ulcers, gastritis, hepatosplenomegaly, hypersplenism
Musculoskeletal	Myalgias, arthralgias, osteoporosis, pathologic fractures
Reproductive	Uterine cramping
Hematopoietic	Lymphadenopathy, bleeding disorders, cytopenia, recurrent infections

Data from Refs.[3,5–7,10,12–14,17–22]

DIAGNOSIS
Overview of Diagnostic Tests

The following tests may be useful as part of a mastocytosis diagnostic evaluation.

Bone marrow biopsy
Bone marrow biopsy is performed to make a diagnosis of systemic mastocystosis, as discussed later.

Skin biopsy
A skin biopsy is crucial to confirm a diagnosis of CM.[5]

Total tryptase level
Tryptase is a marker of mast cell degranulation released in parallel with histamine and is typically elevated in those with SM.[23,24] Patients with CM often have normal levels of total tryptase. In children with CM, however, elevated serum baseline tryptase may predict an increased risk of anaphylaxis. One study found that children with tryptase levels greater than 6 ng/mL are more likely to require daily treatment to manage symptoms and prevent severe episodes, and those with levels greater than 15.5 ng/mL were at risk for hospitalization.[25] The total tryptase level in serum or plasma seems to be a more discriminating biomarker than urinary methylhistamine for a diagnosis of SM.[26] As discussed previously, total tryptase values are recommended by the WHO as a minor criterion for use in the diagnostic evaluation of SM.

Complete blood cell count with differential
In SM, complete blood cell counts may reveal anemia, thrombocytopenia, thrombocytosis, leukocytosis, and eosinophilia as well as abnormal forms, because advanced forms of SM can be associated with other hematologic malignancies.[9]

Blood smear
A blood smear can be done to evaluate for possible associated hematologic malignancies.

Plasma or urinary histamine level
Although not routinely ordered, patients with mastocytosis often have elevated 24-hour urine histamine levels. Compared with total tryptase level, urine or plasma histamine seems a less specific biomarker for the diagnosis of SM.[26]

Serum chemistry panel
Serum chemistry panel with SM is used to monitor for liver involvement and electrolyte imbalances.

Regular bone densitometry
Regular bone densitometry for patients with SM is used to screen for and monitor osteopenia or osteoporosis.

Abdominal ultrasound
Abdominal ultrasound can be useful to evaluate for organomegaly with SM.[5]

Diagnosis of Systemic Mastocytosis

For SM, the preferred method of diagnosing is via bone marrow biopsy. The WHO has established the following criteria for diagnosing SM.[9,27]

Major criterion
Multifocal dense infiltrates of mast cells (>15 in aggregate) in tryptase-stained biopsy sections of the bone marrow or of another extracutaneous organ.

Minor criterion

1. In biopsy of bone marrow or other extracutaneous organ(s), more than 25% of the mast cells show abnormal morphology (ie, are atypical mast cell type I or are spindle shaped) in multifocal lesions In histologic examination.
2. A point mutation at codon 816 in the KIT receptor gene may be detected in bone marrow, blood, or other internal organ.
3. KIT-positive mast cells in bone marrow, blood, or other internal organs are found to express CD2 and/or CD25.
4. Serum total tryptase level persistently is greater than 20 ng/mL. (Note: this criterion cannot be used if a patient has an AHNMD disorder.)

   *** The presence of 1 major and 1 minor criteria or 3 minor criteria constitute a diagnosis of SM.

Diagnosis of the different mastocytosis categories
Indolent systemic mastocytosis A majority of adult patients with SM are in the ISM category.[28] These patients fit the criteria for SM and may have an enlarged liver or spleen. The gastrointestinal (GI) tract also may be affected. Mediator-related symptoms are common, but the grade of bone marrow infiltration is low, usually less than 5%.[28] In most patients, the serum tryptase concentration exceeds 20 ng/mL, but a normal level of tryptase does not rule out either mastocytosis or another mast cell activation disorder.[28]

Systemic mastocytosis with associated clonal hematologic non–mast cell lineage disease Patients with SM with AHNMD fit the WHO criteria for SM AND myelodysplastic syndrome, myeloproliferative syndrome, acute myeloid leukemia, or non-Hodgkin lymphoma.[28] These patients often do not have urticaria pigmentosa–like skin lesions.

Agressive systemic mastocytosis In the rare disorder, ASM, patients fit the criteria for SM, and their bone marrow biopsy reveals abnormal blood cell formation that does not fit the diagnostic criteria for myelodysplastic syndrome, myeloproliferative syndrome, acute myeloid leukemia, or non-Hodgkin lymphoma.[28] The prognosis and clinical course of patients with ASM is variable, with some patients experiencing a rapidly declining course over 1 to 2 years, whereas others follow a slower course with several years of survival.[28]

Mast cell leukemia MCL is rare and those with this diagnosis fit the criteria for SM and the presence of greater than or equal to 20% atypical mast cells in the marrow or greater than or equal to 10% in the blood; however, an aleukemic variant is frequently encountered in which the number of circulating mast cells is less than 10%.[29] The shape of mast cells and their nuclei have malignant features. Patients with MCL have an overall poor prognosis. Progression to multiple organ failure with weight loss, bone pain, and organomegaly develops over weeks to months, with death usually occurring within 12 to 24 months of diagnosis.[29,30]

Diagnosis of Cutaneous Mastocytosis

Approximately two-thirds of cases of CM occur in children. CM is diagnosed by the presence of typical skin lesions that demonstrate the Darier sign and a positive skin biopsy demonstrating characteristic clusters of mast cells. A Darier sign is demonstrated when the skin lesion of CM becomes raised and erythematous and itches when it is rubbed briskly. Patients with CM do not fulfill diagnostic criteria for SM (as discussed previously) and show no evidence of organ involvement other than the skin.[24,31] Rarely, CM can present with acute mast cell activation events, including anaphylaxis.

There are 3 types of cutaneous mastocytosis.

1. Urticaria pigmentosa, also known as maculopapular CM, is the most common form of mastocytosis in adults and children, representing 70% to 90% of cases.[5]
2. Diffuse CM (DCM) is rare but can present with more severe symptoms. DCM accounts for 1% to 3% of the cases of CM and can involve the whole skin with the central region and scalp most affected. DCM can appear at birth (congenital and neonatal) or in early infancy. Blistering and bullae may be the presenting symptoms and the blisters can be hemorrhagic.[5]
3. Solitary mastocytoma (mastocytoma of skin) is the second most common form of childhood-onset CM, accounting for approximately 10% to 15% of cases. It often develops before 1 year of age, with most cases presenting within the first 3 months of life; adult involvement is rare.[32]

Other Mastocytosis Diagnostic Categories

Mast cell sarcoma

Mast cell sarcoma (MCS) is a unifocal mast cell tumor with no evidence or criteria for SM and no other skin lesions. There is a destructive growth pattern and high-grade cytology.[33] Systemic involvement is not found among patients at diagnosis of MCS, but generalization with extension to various organs and hematopoietic tissues may occur and even lead to MCL.[9]

Extracutaneous mastocytoma

Extracutaneous mastocytoma is a unifocal mast cell tumor with no evidence or criteria for SM and no other skin lesions. There is a nondestructive growth pattern and low-grade cytology.[9]

MASTOCYTOSIS TREATMENT
Trigger Avoidance

Patients with SM should be counseled that various exposures and situations can trigger symptoms and should avoid exposures that trigger or aggravate their symptoms to the extent possible. These exposures may include heat, humidity, cold, emotional stress, strenuous exercise, alcohol, spicy food, infections, vaccinations, anesthesia, surgery, medications, and endoscopic procedures and lack of sleep. Insect stings can precipitate symptoms in patients with mastocytosis, even when there is no IgE-mediated venom allergy detectable by skin or blood testing. In infants and children, symptoms can be induced or aggravated by mood (anger or irritability), fever, skin abrasion, or rubbing, and teething can induce symptoms.[25] There are various medications that may cause mast cell activation in patients with both CM and SM. Therefore, if possible, the following medications should be avoided: opioids, vancomycin, aspirin and other NSAIDS, radiocontrast agents, thiamine, quinine, and succinylcholine.[34–36]

Anaphylaxis Treatment

The incidence of anaphylaxis is much higher in those with mastocytosis.[18,37] All patients and caretakers should be taught how to recognize and treat anaphylaxis and carry an epinephrine autoinjector. Hymenoptera stings, in particular, are prone to cause anaphylaxis in patients with mastocytosis.[38] All patients with reactions to hymenoptera stings should be evaluated with skin tests or in vitro tests for venom-specific IgE, and those testing positive should be offered venom immunotherapy to reduce the risk of anaphylaxis on subsequent stings. Venom immunotherapy is effective to treat IgE-mediated hymenoptera anaphylaxis in patients with mastocytosis. Its use is recommended despite a high risk of adverse reactions during the build-up phase because it provides protection from anaphylaxis in approximately three-quarters of the patients.[39] The risk:benefit ratio for immunotherapy with hymenoptera venom favors immunotherapy, because patients with mastocytosis can suffer severe anaphylaxis in response to an hymenoptera sting, including fatalities even with epinephrine treatment.[38] Pretreatment with omalizumab may reduce the risk of systemic reactions to venom immunotherapy for those with mastocytosis, but it is not currently approved for this use in the United States.[40]

Mastocytosis patients with recurrent anaphylaxis should be treated with maximized doses of antimediator agents (maximal doses of H_1-antihistamines and H_2-antihistamines and antileukotriene drugs). In patients unresponsive to antimediator therapy, low-dose maintenance glucocorticoids or cytoreductive measures (interferon [IFN] alpha, cladribine, omalizumab, or tyrosine kinase inhibitor, depending on c-kit mutational status) can be considered.[41]

SYMPTOM-SPECIFIC TREATMENT

There is no curative therapy for mastocytosis. Therefore, treatment is intended to reduce the following symptoms and improve quality of life.[42]

See **Table 4** for a list of treatments of cutaneous symptoms.

Treatment of Gastrointestinal Symptoms

Oral cromolyn can help treat GI symptoms, such as diarrhea and abdominal pain, nausea, and vomiting.[45]

Table 4
Treatment of cutaneous symptoms

Medication	Indicated for
Topical steroids or intralesion steroid injections	Topical or intralesional steroids can be used for cutaneous lesions that involve a limited body area. Systemic corticosteroids can be used with severe skin disease.
Psoralen–UV-A photochemotherapy	Cutaneous lesions
H₁-antihistamines	Pruritus, flushing
Leukotriene receptor antagonists (montelukast and zafirlukast)	Flushing, and itching in patients unresponsive to H₁-antihistamines
Oral cromolyn (FDA approved for mastocytosis)	Pruritus, whealing, and flushing
Aspirin (up to 650 mg twice daily)	Helps with flushing, if the patient is known to tolerate NSAIDs

Data from Refs.[43–45]

H_2-antihistamines (cimetidine, ranitidine, and famotidine) and proton pump inhibitors may be used to treat abdominal discomfort and gastroesophageal reflux disease.[9]

Leukotriene receptor antagonists (montelukast and zafirlukast) may help abdominal cramping.[46]

Anticholinergics and menthol can be used to relieve intestinal cramping.

Systemic steroids can be used to help treat malabsorption that can occur with SM.

Treatment of Musculoskeletal Symptoms: Bone Pain, Osteoporosis, and Fractures

Oral cromolyn may help relieve bone pain.

Vitamin D (and calcium) can be supplemented to reduce risk for osteoporosis and fractures.[20]

Spine x-ray and densitometric examinations are recommended to screen for osteoporosis/fractures.

Treatment of Depression

Antidepressants: selective serotonin reuptake inhibitors and tricyclic antidepressants can be used to treat depression in mastocytosis.

Tyrosine kinase therapy may improve depressive symptoms in patients with SM.[47]

Treatment of Lung symptoms

β_2-Agonists can relieve bronchoconstriction that can occur from increased histamine levels.

Inhaled or systemic corticosteroids can treat airway inflammation and associated bronchoconstriction.

Treatment of Ascites

Systemic steroids may be useful in mastocytosis associated ascites.[9] Overall, however, systemic therapy with corticosteroids is often disappointing because the primary mode of action of corticosteroids is redistribution rather than death of mast cells.

Associated Cognitive Disorders

H_1-antihistamines and H_2-antihistamines are considered first-line treatments.[9]

Oral cromolyn is considered second-line treatment of mastocytosis-related cognitive dysfunction.

DIAGNOSIS-SPECIFIC TREATMENT
Treatment of Cutaneous Mastocytosis

There are no therapies that change the natural course of CM and none of the currently available therapeutic measures induces permanent involution of cutaneous or visceral lesions. A few patients with CM may experience a regression of cutaneous lesions without treatment, which can correspond to either improvement or possible progression to systemic disease. Therapy is conservative and aimed at symptom relief because the prognosis for most patients with CM is excellent. The management of CM includes lifestyle modifications, such as the use of lukewarm water for bathing, air conditioning for hot weather, and avoidance of triggers for mast cell degranulation. Patients should be advised to avoid agents that precipitate mediator release, such as NSAIDs, alcohol, and opiates.

Symptomatic therapy for CM involves agents that inhibit the release of mediators or antagonize H_1 and H_2 receptors, such as antihistamines. Skin-targeted therapies aimed at resolution of the lesions of CM are psoralen–UV-A photochemotherapy and topical corticosteroid therapy either by occlusion or intralesional injection for a few lesions.[44] Risks of skin cancer increases, however, with repeated psoralen–UV-A photochemotherapy, if more than 200 treatments are required.[48] H_1-antihistamines and H_2-antihistamines can be used to decrease pruritus, flushing, and GI symptoms. Nifedipine, a calcium channel blocker, may inhibit cold-induced urtication and flushing in patients with CM but is not Food and Drug Administration (FDA) approved for treatment of mastocytosis.[49] Treatment selection is made on the basis of clinical manifestations, onset of disease, probability of spontaneous involution, and severity of CM and SM symptoms.[44] Future novel therapy for CM includes immune modulators, such as imatinib. One successful case report from 2008 described successful treatment of disease symptoms and progression with imatinib.[50]

Treatment of Systemic Mastocytosis

SM has no known cure and tends to be progressive.[42] The treatment algorithm for SM is complex, and the condition is primarily managed by a hematologist. Patients with advanced forms should be referred to centers with expertise in SM. The mainstay of treatment of most categories of mastocytosis is H_1-antihistamines and H_2-antihistamines with the addition of corticosteroids for more severe symptoms. Commonly used H_1-antihistamines include oral cetirizine, fexofenadine, hydroxyzine, or doxepin and commonly used H_2 blockers include ranitidine, cimetidine, and famotidine.[43] Other commonly used treatments for SM include corticosteroids, leukotriene inhibitors, cromolyn, and IFN. Pharmacotherapies may be needed for patients with any subtype of SM, although symptoms arising from mediator release are most prominent in patients with ISM and ASM.

Although most patients have the indolent variant of SM, in which intensive therapy is not needed, others can suffer from serious disease with aggressive behavior requiring mast cell eradication with cytostatic growth-inhibitory drugs.[51] Among these, IFN alfa and cladribine have shown considerable improvement in symptoms, but none of the treated patients achieved a complete remission.[51] Moreover, both drugs are bone marrow suppressive and cause serious side effects.[51]

Tyrosine kinase inhibitors may be appropriate for some patients with SM. Effective suppression of activated c-kit can result in killing of KIT-mutated mast cells and improvement in SM symptoms.[16,52] Tyrosine kinase inhibitors, however, vary in their ability to act on wild-type or mutated molecules. Imatinib is a tyrosine kinase inhibitor approved by the FDA for use in patients with ASM with organ dysfunction due to progressive infiltration of various organs by mast cells without D816V c-kit mutation or unknown c-kit mutation status.[53] Unfortunately, most patients with SM are not candidates for imatinib (Gleevec) therapy because they have the D816V KIT mutation, which confers resistance to imatinib.[54] Other tyrosine kinase inhibitors that have been administered to patients with SM include masitinib, and dasatinib. Masitinib is a promising treatment of indolent forms of SM,[55] but clinical trials with dasatinib have not yielded significant improvements.[56,57]

Allogeneic hematopoietic cell transplantation has been performed in a few patients with advanced forms of SM but it is not appropriate for indolent or cutaneous forms of mastocytosis.[58] Other possible treatments for SM include calcineurin inhibitors, such as pimecrolimus.[59]

Treatment of Indolent Systemic Mastocytosis

Treatment of ISM is intended to prevent mast cell mediator release and is mainly symptomatic.[9,60] ISM progresses slowly or not at all and most patients have normal life expectancy. Therefore, therapies to reduce mast cell numbers, which are associated with significant adverse effects, are generally not indicated or recommended. Treatment usually includes mediator-targeting drugs, including antihistamines, but does not usually require cytoreductive agents, except for considering IFN-2b for severe osteoporosis.[9,60]

SYSTEMIC MASTOCYTOSIS WITH ASSOCIATED CLONAL HEMATOLOGIC NON–MAST CELL LINEAGE DISEASE

Treatment of patients with SM-AHNMD depends on the associated hematologic condition. Generally, the approach is to treat AHNMD as if SM were not present and to treat the mastocytosis as if the AHNMD were not present. Successful treatment of the hematologic disorder has not been shown to change or improve their SM. The prognosis of patients with SM-AHNMD is that of the hematologic disorder present.

Treatment of Agressive Systemic Mastocytosis

ASM is a clonal mast cell disease characterized by progressive growth of neoplastic cells in diverse organs but most frequently affected are the bone marrow, skeletal system, liver, spleen, and the GI tract. Respective clinical findings (so called C-findings) include cytopenias, osteolysis (or osteoporosis) with pathologic fractures, hepatosplenomegaly with impaired liver function and ascites, and malabsorption. During the past decade, several treatment strategies for ASM have been proposed. One promising approach may be combination treatment with IFN alpha and glucocorticoids.[61,62]

The most commonly administered therapies are IFN alpha-2b, cladribine, glucocorticoids, tyrosine kinase inhibitors, and hydroxyurea. Cladribine is often reserved for patients who do not respond to IFN alpha. Prophylaxis to prevent Pneumocystis jiroveci pneumonia is suggested for at least 3 months after therapy is complete and until the CD4 count is greater than 200/μL. Orally administered glucocorticoids are helpful for patients with ASM and severe malabsorption or ascites and can be given as a 2-week to 3-week taper, although some patients may require low-dose maintenance therapy.

In patients with ASM, IFN alfa (with or without corticosteroids) can control dermatologic, hematological, GI, skeletal, and mediator-release symptoms but may be poorly tolerated. Cladribine has broad therapeutic activity, particularly when rapid debulking is indicated; the main toxicity is myelosuppression. Imatinib has a therapeutic role in the presence of an imatinib-sensitive KIT mutation or in patients with unmutated *KITD816*.[28] Imatinib is approved by the FDA for ASM in patients who do not have a D816V KIT mutation or those with unknown mutational status. Splenectomy may be indicated for hypersplenism in association with severe anemia and thrombocytopenia.[63]

Hydroxyurea has also been administered to patients with ASM and SM-AHNMD, mainly for the treatment of associated myeloproliferative disorders, although there are few published data on efficacy.

Hydroxyurea has few side effects compared with other chemotherapeutic agents, although hematologic toxicity and GI side effects may be problematic at higher doses. Patients should use contraception because hydroxyurea is a teratogen.

Mast Cell Leukemia

There is no approved standard therapy for MCL. There are few options are available for treatment and, because of the rarity of the disease, few clinical trials address the question.[29] Patients with MCL are often treated with polychemotherapy, similarly to those with acute leukemia. Administered agents have included cladribine, tyrosine kinase inhibitors, and polychemotherapy. Bone marrow transplantation may be considered, although sustained remission has not been reported.[29] Patients with MCL are particularly prone to GI bleeding due to heparin release from the high number of mast cells present and possibly associated coagulopathies,[64] and chronic proton pump inhibitor therapy should be considered for GI prophylaxis. Therapy usually fails and the median survival time is less than 6 months.

Mast Cell Sarcoma

MCS is an extremely rare and aggressive subtype of mastocytosis with poor prognosis. MCS is an aggressive tumor that exhibits an always fatal evolution despite various classic polychemotherapies with or without radiotherapy. The median survival is only 12 months, and no good treatment is available.[29]

Extracutaneous Mastocytoma

Treatment is surgical for extracuteneous mastocytomas, although they are extremely uncommon and prognosis is unknown due to its rarity.[65]

REFERENCES

1. Horny HP, Sotlar K, Valent P. Mastocytosis: state of the art. Pathobiology 2007;74: 121–32.
2. Metcalfe D. Mast cells and mastocytosis. Blood 2008;112(4):946–56.
3. Gulen T, Hagglund H, Dahlen B, et al. Mascytosis: the puzzling clinical spectrum and challenging diagnostic aspects of an enigmatic disease. J Intern Med 2015; 279(3):211–28.
4. Valent P, Akin C, Wolfgang S, et al. Mastocytosis: pathology, genetics and current options for therapy. Leuk Lymphoma 2005;46(1):35–48.
5. Castells M, Metcalfe D, Escribano L. Guidelines for the diagnosis and treatment of cutaneous mastocytosis in children. Am J Clin Dermatol 2011;12(4):259–70.

6. Magliacane D, Parente R, Triggiani M. Current concepts on diagnosis and treatment of mastocytosis. Transl Med UniSa 2014;8(8):65–74.
7. Maluf LC, Barros JA, Macho Filho CD. Mastocytosis. An Bras Dermatol 2009; 84(3):213–25.
8. Valent P. Mastocytosis: a paradigmatic example of a rare disease with complex biology and pathology. Am J Cancer Res 2013;3:159–72.
9. Pardanani A. Systemic mastocytosis in adults: 2015 update on diagnosis, risk stratification, and management. Am J Hematol 2015;90(3):250–62.
10. Metcalfe DD. Regulation of normal and neoplastic human mast cell development in mastocytosis. Trans Am Clin Climatol Assoc 2005;116:185–204.
11. Abraham SN, St John AL. Mast cell-orchestrated immunity to pathogens. Nat Rev Immunol 2010;10:440–52.
12. Theoharides TC, Valent P, Akin C. Mast cells, mastocytosis, and related disorders. N Engl J Med 2015;373:163–72.
13. Brockow K, Jofer C, Behrendt H, et al. Anaphylaxis in patients with mastocystosis: a study on history, clinical feature and risk factors in 120 patients. Allergy 2008;63:226–32.
14. Bonadonna P, Lombardo C, Zanotti R. Mastocytosis and allergic disease. J Investig Allergol Clin Immunol 2014;24(5):288–97.
15. Kitamura Y, Go S. Decreased production of mast cells in S1/S1^d mice. Blood 1979;53:492–7.
16. Akin C, Metcalfe DD. The biology of Kit in disease and the application of pharmacogenetics. J Allergy Clin Immunol 2004;114:13–9.
17. McNeill O, Katelaris CH. Mastocytosis-where are we now? World Allergy Organization; 2011.
18. Greenhawt M, Akin C. Mastocytosis and allergy. Curr Opin Allergy Clin Immunol 2007;7(5):387–92.
19. Bot I, Biessen EA. Mast cells in atherosclerosis. Thromb Haemost 2011;106(5): 820–6.
20. Rossini M, Zanotti R, Bonadonna P, et al. Bone mineral density, bone turnover markers and fractures in patients with indolent systemic mastocytosis. Bone 2011;49(4):880.
21. Stein JA, Kamino H, Walters RF, et al. Mastocytosis with urticaria pigmentosa and osteoporosis. Dermatol Online J 2008;14(10):2.
22. Lawrence JB, Friedman BS, Travis WD, et al. Hematologic manifsestations of systemic mast cell disease: a prospective study of laboratory and morphologic features and their relation to prognosis. Am J Med 1991;91:612.
23. Valent P. Diagnostic evaluation and classification of mastocytosis. Immunol Allergy Clin North Am 2006;26(3):515–34.
24. Patnaik MM, Rindos M, Kouides PA, et al. Systemic mastocytosis: a concise clinical and laboratory review. Arch Pathol Lab Med 2007;131(5):784–91.
25. Barnes M, Van L, DeLong L, et al. Severity of cutaneous findings predict the presence of systemic symptoms in pediatric maculopapular cutaneous mastocytosis. Pediatr Dermatol 2014;31(3):271–5.
26. Schwartz LB. Diagnostic value of tryptase in anaphylaxis and mastocytosis. Immunol Allergy Clin North Am 2006;26(3):451–63.
27. Sánchez-Muñoz L, Alvarez-Twose I, García-Montero AC, et al. Evaluation of the WHO criteria for the classification of patients with mastocytosis. Mod Pathol 2011;24(9):1157–68.
28. Pardanani A. Systemic mastocytosis in adults: 2012 Update on diagnosis, risk stratification, and management. Am J Hematol 2012;87(4):401–11.

29. Georgin-Lavialle S, Lhermitte L, Dubreuil P, et al. Mast cell leukemia. Blood 2013; 121(8):1285–95.

30. Valent P, Sperr WR, Schwartz LB, et al. Diagnosis and classification of mast cell proliferative disorders: delineation from immunologic diseases and non-mast cell hematopoietic neoplasms. J Allergy Clin Immunol 2004;114(1):3.

31. Johnson M, Verstovsek S, Jorgensen J, et al. Utility of the World Heath Organization classification criteria for the diagnosis of systemic mastocytosis in bone marrow. Mod Pathol 2009;22(1):50–7.

32. Semenov Y. Persistent solitary lesion in an 8-month-old boy. Contemp Pediatr 2013.

33. Georgin-Lavialle S, Aguilar C, Guieze R, et al. Mast cell sarcoma: a rare and aggressive entity–report of two cases and review of the literature. J Clin Oncol 2013;31(6):e90–7.

34. Deverrière G, Carré D, Nae I, et al. Bullous mastocytosis in infancy: a rare presentation. Arch Pediatr 2012;19(7):722–5.

35. Guyer AC, Saff RR, Conroy M, et al. Comprehensive allergy evaluation is useful in the subsequent care of patients with drug hypersensitivity reactions during anesthesia. J Allergy Clin Immunol Pract 2015;3(1):94–100.

36. Hepner DL, Castells MC. Anaphylaxis during the perioperative period. Anesth Analg 2003;97(5):1381–95.

37. Akin C, Fumo G, Yavuz AS, et al. A novel form of mastocytosis associated with a transmembrane c-kit mutation and response to imatinib. Blood 2004;103(8):3222.

38. Ruëff F, Placzek M, Przybilla B. Mastocytosis and Hymenoptera venom allergy. Curr Opin Allergy Clin Immunol 2006;6(4):284.

39. González de Olano D, Alvarez-Twose I, Esteban-López MI, et al. Safety and effectiveness of immunotherapy in patients with indolent systemic mastocytosis presenting with Hymenoptera venom anaphylaxis. J Allergy Clin Immunol 2008; 121(2):519.

40. Kontou-Fili K, Filis CI. Prolonged high-dose omalizumab is required to control reactions to venom immunotherapy in mastocytosis. Allergy 2009;64(9):1384.

41. Jagdis A, Vadas P. Omalizumab effectively prevents recurrent refractory anaphylaxis in a patient with monoclonal mast cell activation syndrome. Ann Allergy Asthma Immunol 2014;113(1):115–6.

42. Hennessy B, Giles F, Cortes J, et al. Management of patients with systemic mastocytosis: review of M. D. Anderson Cancer Center experience. Am J Hematol 2004;77(3):209.

43. Worobec AS. Treatment of systemic mast cell disorders. Hematol Oncol Clin North Am 2000;14(3):659.

44. Wolff K. Treatment of cutaneous mastocytosis. Int Arch Allergy Immunol 2002; 127(2):156–9.

45. Horan RF, Sheffer AL, Austen KF. Cromolyn sodium in the management of systemic mastocytosis. J Allergy Clin Immunol 1990;85(5):852.

46. Tolar J, Tope WD, Neglia JP. Leukotriene-receptor inhibition for the treatment of systemic mastocytosis. N Engl J Med 2004;350(7):735.

47. Moura DS, Sultan S, Georgin-Lavialle S, et al. Depression in patients with mastocytosis: prevalence, features and effects of masitinib therapy. PLoS One 2011; 6(10):e26375.

48. Kinsler VA, Hawk JL, Atherton DJ. Diffuse cutaneous mastocytosis treated with psoralen photochemotherapy: case report and review of the literature. Br J Dermatol 2005;152(1):179–80.

49. Fairley JA, Pentland AP, Voorhees JJ. Urticaria pigmentosa responsive to nifedipine. J Am Acad Dermatol 1984;11(4 Pt 2):740–3.
50. Hoffmann KM, Moser A, Lohse P, et al. Successful treatment of progressive cutaneous mastocytosis with imatinib in a 2-year-old boy carrying a somatic KIT mutation. Blood 2008;112(5):1655–7.
51. Kluin-Nelemans HC, Ferenc V, van Doormaal JJ, et al. Lenalidomide therapy in systemic mastocytosis. Leuk Res 2009;33(3):e19–22.
52. Longley BJ, Ma Y, Carter E, et al. New approaches to therapy for mastocytosis. A case for treatment with kit kinase inhibitors. Hematol Oncol Clin North Am 2000; 14(3):689.
53. Bains SN, Hsieh FH. Current approaches to the diagnosis and treatment of systemic mastocytosis. Ann Allergy Asthma Immunol 2010;104(1):1–10 [quiz: 10-2, 41].
54. Vega-Ruiz A, Cortes JE, Sever M, et al. Phase II study of imatinib mesylate as therapy for patients with systemic mastocytosis. Leuk Res 2009;33(11):1481.
55. Paul C, Sans B, Suarez F, et al. Masitinib for the treatment of systemic and cutaneous mastocytosis with handicap: a phase 2a study. Am J Hematol 2010; 85(12):921.
56. Aichberger KJ, Sperr WR, Gleixner KV, et al. Treatment responses to cladribine and dasatinib in rapidly progressing aggressive mastocytosis. Eur J Clin Invest 2008;38(11):869.
57. Verstovsek S, Tefferi A, Cortes J, et al. Phase II study of dasatinib in Philadelphia chromosome-negative acute and chronic myeloid diseases, including systemic mastocytosis. Clin Cancer Res 2008;14(12):3906.
58. Ustun C, Reiter A, Scott BL, et al. Hematopoietic stem-cell transplantation for advanced systemic mastocytosis. J Clin Oncol 2014;32(29):3264–74.
59. Ma Z, Jiao Z. Mast cells as targets of pimecrolimus. Curr Pharm Des 2011;17(34): 3823–9.
60. Pardanani A. How I treat patients with indolent and smoldering mastocytosis (rare conditions but difficult to manage). Blood 2013;121:3085–94.
61. Valent P, Akin C, Sperr WR, et al. Aggressive systemic mastocytosis and related mast cell disorders: current treatment options and proposed response criteria. Leuk Res 2003;27(7):635–41.
62. Valent P, Sperr W, Akin C. How I treat patients with advanced systemic mastocytosis. Blood 2010;116(26):5812–7.
63. Friedman B, Darling G, Norton J, et al. Splenectomy in the management of systemic mast cell disease. Surgery 1990;107:94.
64. Carvalhosa AB, Aouba A, Damaj G, et al. A French national survey on clotting disorders in mastocytosis. Medicine (Baltimore) 2015;94(40):e1414.
65. Castells MC. Extracutaneous mastocytoma. J Allergy Clin Immunol 2006;117(6): 1513.

Complementary and Alternative Treatment for Allergic Conditions

Juan Qiu, MD, PhD[a],*, Kristen Grine, DO[b]

KEYWORDS

- Complementary and alternative medicine • Traditional Chinese medicine
- Acupuncture • Homeopathy • Asthma • Allergic rhinitis • Atopic dermatitis
- Allergies

KEY POINTS

- Complementary and alternative medicine (CAM) is increasingly utilized in the western countries for allergic conditions despite the paucity of conclusive study results.
- Several CAM modalities have showed promising therapeutic efficacy in allergic conditions, although the mechanisms of action are still largely unclear.
- Clinicians should be familiar with these therapies in advising patients about the alternative treatment options for allergic conditions.

INTRODUCTION

Complementary and alternative medicine (CAM) is any therapeutic intervention outside the realm of conventional allopathic medicine. Although CAM is commonly used by 80% of the world's population, its utilization is growing in western countries and has increased to near 50% of the US population in 2015. Given this increasing prevalence, it is essential that clinicians have the resources and knowledge to advise their patients in the utilization, benefits, and potential adverse effects of these alternative therapies.

More than 20% of the US population suffers from allergic disorders, which include asthma, allergic rhinitis, and atopic dermatitis. Epidemiologic data in patients with allergic disorders indicate that 42% of people have used CAM for these conditions.[1,2] This increase in popularity of CAM for allergic conditions is largely due to the reputed

No conflict of interest.
[a] Department of Family and Community Medicine, Pennsylvania State University College of Medicine, Penn State Hershey Medical Group, 32 Colonnade Way, State College, PA 16803, USA; [b] Department of Family and Community Medicine, Pennsylvania State University College of Medicine, Penn State Hershey Medical Group, 476 Rolling Ridge Drive, #101, State College, PA 16801, USA
* Corresponding author.
E-mail address: jqiu@hmc.psu.edu

Prim Care Clin Office Pract 43 (2016) 519–526
http://dx.doi.org/10.1016/j.pop.2016.04.012   **primarycare.theclinics.com**

effectiveness, low cost, and favorable safety profiles of CAM. It is also related to the unsatisfactory results of many conventional therapies, concerns about adverse effects of synthetic drugs, and the paucity of preventive or curative therapies for these chronic diseases. In this article, several CAM therapies for allergic conditions are discussed based on results of randomized controlled trials.

Traditional Chinese Medicine Formula for Asthma

Traditional Chinese medicine (TCM) views allergic disease as resulting from the loss of homeostasis in interactions between human organs, such as the lungs, skin, and gut, with the environment, and foods. TCM practice focuses on establishing and maintaining the balance of yin–yang (2 opposite, but complementary forces), the homeostasis of organ systems in the body, and interactions with the environment. A Chinese herbal formulation is a mixture of many herbs.

Chinese herbs have been used for centuries in Asia to treat asthma. There is increasing scientific evidence to support the use of TCM herbal therapy for asthma. There have been many randomized trials of TCM herbal formulas for asthma,[3] including modified Mai Men Dong Tang (mMMDT),[4] STA-1,[5] and antiasthma herbal medicine intervention (ASHMI).[6,7] ASHMI has received investigational new drug approval in the United States (**Table 1**).

Table 1
Traditional Chinese medicine formula for asthma

TCM Formula	Mechanism of Action	Evidence of Efficacy	Adverse Effects
ASHMI	• Blocking the IgE-mediated early phase airway response, airway hyper-reactivity, pulmonary inflammation, and airway remodeling[8,9] • Reducing histamine and leukotriene release modulates airway smooth muscle contraction associated with increased prostaglandin I2, a potent muscle relaxer[8]	• In 2 randomized trials, ASHMI was found nearly equivalent to oral or inhaled steroid in improving forced expiratory volume in 1 second (FEV1) and peak expiratory flow values, as well as reducing symptoms and inhaled beta 2-agonist use in patients with moderate-to-severe asthma[6] • The improvement in symptom scores, particularly nasal symptoms, was greater in the ASHMI group than in the steroid group	Gastric discomfort[7]
mMMDT	• Affecting steroid metabolism (licorice) and • Immunomodulatory effects (ginseng)[4]	Studies in atopic children with mild-to-moderate persistent asthma[4] showed significant improvements in FEV1 and asthma symptom scores	No
STA-1	Anti-inflammatory and antiallergic properties	Patients treated with STA-1 had improved symptoms scores, increased lung function (FEV1), less systemic glucocorticoid treatment, and decreased total and dust mite-specific IgE compared with baseline[5]	No

Data from Refs.[4–9]

Traditional Chinese Medicine Formula for Allergic Rhinitis

A systematic review of randomized controlled trials of TCM remedies for allergic rhinitis showed that TCM reduced nasal symptom scores relative to placebo with no serious adverse effects.[10] However, the published trials are generally small, and further studies are needed before firm conclusions can be drawn[11] (**Table 2**).

Traditional Chinese Medicine Formula for Atopic Dermatitis

Oral and topical preparations of TCM have been used for centuries in Asia for the treatment of atopic dermatitis. Nonetheless, there are only a few randomized controlled trials evaluating their efficacy. A Cochrane review in 2015 did not find conclusive evidence that Chinese Herbal Medicine (CHM) taken by mouth or applied topically to the skin could reduce the severity of atopic dermatitis in children or adults[14] (**Table 3**).

Traditional Chinese Medicine Formula for Food Allergy

Food allergy affects as many as 8% of young children and 5% of adults.[20] The standard of care for food allergy management includes strict avoidance and immediate access to rescue medications. Currently, there is no effective therapy or cure.

Food Allergy Herbal Formula-2 (FAHF-2), a TCM formula, is the first botanic investigational new drug approved for clinical studies for food allergy by the US Food and Drug Administration (FDA). Murine model studies and phase I trials have demonstrated that this formula is safe and well tolerated by subjects with peanut, tree nut, fish, and/or shellfish allergy.[21,22] A recent multicenter, randomized, double-blind, placebo-controlled phase II clinical trial showed that FAHF-2 is a safe herbal medication for subjects with food allergy. However, efficacy for improving tolerance to food allergens was not demonstrated at the dose and duration used.[23] This study was limited by poor drug adherence. The mechanism of action of FAHF-2 is unclear.

Herbal Therapies for Allergic Rhinitis and Conjunctivitis

Various herbal remedies may be used by patients for allergic rhinitis and conjunctivitis. Several of them have showed encouraging evidence as effective treatment options, although scientific evaluation of herbal products has been limited[24] (**Table 4**).

Table 2
Traditional Chinese medicine formula for allergic rhinitis

TCM Formula	Mechanism of Action	Evidence of Efficacy	Adverse Effects
Xin Yi San (XYS)	Suppressing serum IgE levels and IgE specific to dust mites[12]	Reduction in nasal congestion, sneeze and rhinorrhea, decrease in nasal airway resistance, and increase in the nostril area compared with placebo in a randomized double-blind placebo control trial.[12]	No
Allergic Rhinitis Nasal formulation (ARND)	Unclear	Improving overall nasal symptoms with greatest improvement of sleep quality, appetite, and overall joy[13]	No

Data from Yang S, Yu C, Chen Y, et al. Traditional Chinese medicine, Xin-yi-san, reduces nasal symptoms of patients with perennial allergic rhinitis by its diverse immunomodulatory effects. Int Immunopharmacol 2010;10:951; and Chui SH, Shek SL, Fong MY, et al. A panel study to evaluate quality of life assessments in patients suffering from allergic rhinitis after treatment with a Chinese herbal nasal drop. Phytother Res 2010;24:609.

Table 3
Traditional Chinese medicine formula for atopic dermatitis

TCM Formula	Mechanism of Action	Evidence of Efficacy	Adverse Effects
PentaHerbs	Inhibiting inflammatory mediator release from mast cells[15]	• Improved quality of life and reduced topical corticosteroid use[16] • No significant difference in extent and severity of the disease compared with placebo in a randomized trial[17]	No
Xiao-Feng-San (XFS)	Unclear	Showed significantly greater improvement in the total lesion, erythema, surface damage, pruritus, and sleep scores in the treatment group compared with placebo in a randomized trial[18]	No
Pei Tu Qing Xin Tang (PTQXT)	Unclear	Significantly decreased the extent and severity of allergic dermatitis compared with control for patients with moderate to severe allergic dermatitis in a randomized control study[19]	No

Data from Refs.[15–19]

Other Nasal Sprays, Powders, and Ointments for Allergic Rhinitis

Nasal sprays containing either dilute capsaicin or inert cellulose and petrolatum-based ointment have demonstrated efficacy in randomized controlled trials (**Table 5**).

Table 4
Herbal therapies for allergic rhinitis and conjunctivitis

Herb Name	Mechanism of Action	Evidence of Efficacy	Side Effects
Butterbur (Petasites hybridus)	Possibly by altering the leukotriene pathway[25]	In a systematic review, butterbur compared favorably with 10 mg of cetirizine and 180 mg of fexofenadine[24]	Hepatic toxicity
Tinofend (Tinospora cordifolia)	Unclear	Significantly improved nasal symptoms compared with placebo in a double-blind randomized trial[26]	Leukocytosis and hepatic toxicity
Aller-7 (mix of 7 Indian herbs)	• Antihistaminic and • Anti-inflammatory properties	In a randomized trial, Aller-7 appeared to be equivalent to cetirizine in improving nasal symptoms[26]	Mild gastric discomfort and dry mouth
Cinnamon bark, Spanish needle, and acerola	Inhibiting the production of prostaglandin D2[27]	Reduced nasal and eye symptoms[27]	No
Benifuuki green tea	Suppressing the seasonal increase in peripheral blood eosinophil[16]	Decreased the allergy symptoms and improved quality of life[16]	No

Data from Refs.[16,24–27]

Table 5
Other nasal sprays, powders, and ointments for allergic rhinitis

Preparation	Mechanism of Action	Evidence of Efficacy	Adverse Effects
Capsaicin (Capsicum annum)	Proposed to desensitize nasal nerve fibers and reduce nasal hyper responsiveness[28]	Decreased total nasal symptom score, with the greatest improvement in nasal congestion, sinus pain and pressure, and headache in a randomized trial[28]	No
Cellulose powder	Proposed to block mucosal allergen absorption	Reduced total nasal symptom scores without adverse effects in randomized trials[29–31]	No
Allergen-absorbing ointment	Blocking allergen absorption into the nasal mucosa	Improved nasal symptoms scores and quality of life in randomized studies[32,33]	No

Data from Refs.[28–33]

Acupuncture for Allergic Rhinitis

In TCM, a disease is believed to originate from an imbalance of Qi or poor flow of Qi. Acupuncture is a component of TCM that works on the principle of rebalance of Qi, the life energy, thus allow self-healing.

The study of acupuncture is challenging using the standard randomized, double-blinded, placebo-controlled trials. Such study designs are difficult to perform when examining the effect of acupuncture due to the physical nature of the intervention. Therefore, the conclusion from randomized controlled trials may not reflect the true efficacy of acupuncture.

Although randomized controlled trials of acupuncture for allergic rhinitis draw conflicting conclusions,[34] a recent systematic review and meta-analysis suggests that that acupuncture could be a safe and valid treatment option for allergic rhinitis patients.[35]

Despite the study limitations, acupuncture may be a reasonable option for interested patients with relatively mild disease who wish to minimize medication use and find the cost of therapy acceptable. The clinical practice guideline of the American Academy of Otolaryngology in 2015 recommends that clinicians may offer acupuncture for patients with allergic rhinitis who are interested in nonpharmacological treatment.[36]

Homeopathy

Homeopathy has been in practice since 19th century. The principle of homeopathy is that the disease can be attenuated by dilution of substances that cause these symptoms. Most homeopathic preparations begin with a mineral, plant, or animal substance, which is pulverized and mixed with a water-alcohol solution. It then undergoes serial dilutions.

The evidence of efficacy of homeopathy for allergic conditions is mixed overall.[34] The mechanism of action is unclear. However, with a low risk profile, homeopathy may be an alternative option for patients.

Miscellaneous Complementary and Alternative Medicine Therapies

Laser therapy and a variety of other herbal preparations have been suggested for the treatment of allergic rhinitis and conjunctivitis. However, studies have shown minimal evidence of efficacy and are limited by low quality.

SUMMARY/DISCUSSION

Based on the current studies, the clinical efficacy, mechanism of action, and safety of most CAM treatments are largely unclear. Various therapies have demonstrated promising or mixed results. It is important to recognize that there are significant challenges in designing and conducting scientific studies in CAM using the standard randomized placebo-controlled trials for western medicine. For example, CAM therapies are usually individualized for a particular patient with his/her specific disease state; placebo design is problematic for acupuncture treatment, since there is no inert point in a living body; it is difficult to design control treatment when the mechanisms of action of some CAM modality are poorly understood (such as homeopathy). Therefore the conclusions of the study results are often inclusive. It is important that clinicians recognize these pitfalls when advising patients who are interested in alternative therapies.

REFERENCES

1. Available at: www.nccam.nih.gov/health/backgrounds/wholemed.htm. Accessed September 1, 2015.
2. Radix glycyrrhizae. In: WHO monographs on selected medicinal plants, vol. 1. Geneva (Switzerland): World Health Organization; 1999. p. 183.
3. Li XM. Traditional Chinese herbal remedies for asthma and food allergy. J Allergy Clin Immunol 2007;120:25.
4. Hsu CH, Lu CM, Chang TT. Efficacy and safety of modified Mai-Men-Dong-Tang for treatment of allergic asthma. Pediatr Allergy Immunol 2005;16:76.
5. Chang TT, Huang CC, Hsu CH. Clinical evaluation of the Chinese herbal medicine formula STA-1 in the treatment of allergic asthma. Phytother Res 2006;20:342.
6. Wen MC, Wei CH, Hu ZQ, et al. Efficacy and tolerability of anti-asthma herbal medicine intervention in adult patients with moderate–severe allergic asthma. J Allergy Clin Immunol 2005;116:517.
7. Li XM. Complementary and alternative medicine in pediatric allergic disorders. Curr Opin Allergy Clin Immunol 2009;9:161.
8. Zhang T, Srivastava K, Wen MC, et al. Pharmacology and immunological actions of a herbal medicine ASHMI on allergic asthma. Phytother Res 2010;24:1047.
9. Busse PJ, Schofield B, Birmingham N, et al. The traditional Chinese herbal formula ASHMI inhibits allergic lung inflammation in antigen-sensitized and antigen-challenged aged mice. Ann Allergy Asthma Immunol 2010;104:236.
10. Xue CC, Hügel HM, Li CG, et al. Efficacy, chemistry and pharmacology of Chinese herbal medicine for allergic rhinitis. Curr Med Chem 2004;11:1403.
11. Wang S, Tang Q, Qian W, et al. Meta-analysis of clinical trials on traditional Chinese herbal medicine for treatment of persistent allergic rhinitis. Allergy 2012;67:583.
12. Yang S, Yu C, Chen Y, et al. Traditional Chinese medicine, Xin-yi-san, reduces nasal symptoms of patients with perennial allergic rhinitis by its diverse immunomodulatory effects. Int Immunopharmacol 2010;10:951.
13. Chui SH, Shek SL, Fong MY, et al. A panel study to evaluate quality of life assessments in patients suffering from allergic rhinitis after treatment with a Chinese herbal nasal drop. Phytother Res 2010;24:609.
14. Gu S, Yang AW, Xue CC, et al. Chinese herbal medicine for atopic eczema. Cochrane Database Syst Rev 2013;(9):CD008642.
15. Chan BC, Hon KL, Leung PC, et al. Traditional Chinese medicine for atopic eczema: PentaHerbs formula suppresses inflammatory mediators release from mast cells. J Ethnopharmacol 2008;120:85.

16. Masuda S, Maeda-Yamamoto M, Usui S, et al. 'Benifuuki' green tea containing o-methylated catechin reduces symptoms of Japanese cedar pollinosis: a randomized, double-blind, placebo-controlled trial. Allergol Int 2014;63:211.

17. Hon KL, Leung TF, Ng PC, et al. Efficacy and tolerability of a Chinese herbal medicine concoction for treatment of atopic dermatitis: a randomized, double-blind, placebo-controlled study. Br J Dermatol 2007;157:357.

18. Cheng H-M, Chiang L-C, Jan Y-M, et al. The efficacy and safety of a Chinese herbal product (Xiao-Feng-San) for the treatment of refractory atopic dermatitis: a randomized, double-blind, placebo-controlled trial. Int Arch Allergy Immunol 2011;155:141.

19. Liu J, Mo X, Wu D, et al. Efficacy of a Chinese herbal medicine for the treatment of atopic dermatitis: a randomized controlled study. Complement Ther Med 2015; 23:644.

20. Sicherer S, Sampson HA. Food allergy: epidemiology, pathogenesis, diagnosis, and treatment. J Allergy Clin Immunol 2014;133:492.

21. Srivastava KD, Kattan JD, Zou ZM, et al. The Chinese herbal medicine formula FAHF-2 completely blocks anaphylactic reactions in a murine model of peanut allergy. J Allergy Clin Immunol 2005;115:171.

22. Wang J, Patil SP, Yang N, et al. Safety, tolerability, and immunologic effects of a food allergy herbal formula in food allergic individuals: a randomized, double-blinded, placebo-controlled, dose escalation, phase 1 study. Ann Allergy Asthma Immunol 2010;105:75.

23. Wang J, Jones SM, Pongracic JA, et al. Safety, clinical, and immunologic efficacy of a Chinese herbal medicine (Food Allergy Herbal Formula-2) for food allergy. J Allergy Clin Immunol 2015;136(4):962–70.e1.

24. Guo R, Pittler MH, Ernst E. Herbal medicines for the treatment of allergic rhinitis: a systematic review. Ann Allergy Asthma Immunol 2007;99:483.

25. Jackson CM, Lee DK, Lipworth BJ. The effects of butterbur on the histamine and allergen cutaneous response. Ann Allergy Asthma Immunol 2004;92:250.

26. Badar VA, Thawani VR, Wakode PT, et al. Efficacy of Tinospora cordifolia in allergic rhinitis. J Ethnopharmacol 2005;96:445.

27. Corren J, Lemay M, Lin Y, et al. Clinical and biochemical effects of a combination botanical product (ClearGuard) for allergy: a pilot randomized double-blind placebo-controlled trial. Nutr J 2008;7:20.

28. Bernstein JA, Davis BP, Picard JK, et al. A randomized, double-blind, parallel trial comparing capsaicin nasal spray with placebo in subjects with a significant component of nonallergic rhinitis. Ann Allergy Asthma Immunol 2011;107:171.

29. Emberlin JC, Lewis RA. A double blind, placebo-controlled cross over trial of cellulose powder by nasal provocation with Der p1 and Der f1. Curr Med Res Opin 2007;23:2423.

30. Aberg N, Dahl A, Benson M. A nasally applied cellulose powder in seasonal allergic rhinitis (SAR) in children and adolescents; reduction of symptoms and relation to pollen load. Pediatr Allergy Immunol 2011;22:594.

31. Emberlin JC, Lewis RA. A double blind, placebo controlled trial of inert cellulose powder for the relief of symptoms of hay fever in adults. Curr Med Res Opin 2006; 22:275.

32. Schwetz S, Olze H, Melchisedech S, et al. Efficacy of pollen blocker cream in the treatment of allergic rhinitis. Arch Otolaryngol Head Neck Surg 2004;130:979.

33. Geisthoff UW, Blum A, Rupp-Classen M, et al. Lipid-based nose ointment for allergic rhinitis. Otolaryngol Head Neck Surg 2005;133:754.

34. Kern J, Bielory L. Complementary and Alternative Therapy (CAM) in the Treatment of Allergic Rhinitis. Curr Allergy Asthma Rep 2014;14:479.
35. Feng S, Han M, Fan Y, et al. Acupuncture for the treatment of allergic rhinitis: a systematic review and meta-analysis. Am J Rhinol Allergy 2015;29:57.
36. Seidman MD, Gurgel RK, Lin SY, et al. Clinical practice guideline: allergic rhinitis. Otolaryngol Head Neck Surg 2015;152(1 suppl):S1–43.

Moving?

Make sure your subscription moves with you!

To notify us of your new address, find your **Clinics Account Number** (located on your mailing label above your name), and contact customer service at:

Email: journalscustomerservice-usa@elsevier.com

800-654-2452 (subscribers in the U.S. & Canada)
314-447-8871 (subscribers outside of the U.S. & Canada)

Fax number: 314-447-8029

Elsevier Health Sciences Division
Subscription Customer Service
3251 Riverport Lane
Maryland Heights, MO 63043

*To ensure uninterrupted delivery of your subscription, please notify us at least 4 weeks in advance of move.

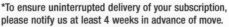

Printed and bound by CPI Group (UK) Ltd, Croydon, CR0 4YY

07/10/2024

01040506-0011